MW00780075

The Natural Body in Somatics Dance Training

The Natural Body in Somatics Dance Training

Doran George

Edited by

Susan Leigh Foster

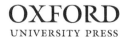
OXFORD
UNIVERSITY PRESS

OXFORD
UNIVERSITY PRESS

Oxford University Press is a department of the University of Oxford. It furthers the University's objective of excellence in research, scholarship, and education by publishing worldwide. Oxford is a registered trade mark of Oxford University Press in the UK and certain other countries.

Published in the United States of America by Oxford University Press
198 Madison Avenue, New York, NY 10016, United States of America.

Library of Congress Control Number: 2020016480
ISBN 978–0–19–753874–6 (pbk.)
ISBN 978–0–19–753873–9 (hbk.)

Hardback printed by Bridgeport National Bindery, Inc., United States of America

Contents

Editor's Note

The loosely coordinated set of regimens known as Somatics emerged over the last half of the twentieth century as a dominant and highly influential training program for cultivating the dancing body. Now installed in the curricula of professional dance schools and university dance programs worldwide, Somatics is regularly envisioned as a central and essential practice for dancers. In many cases it has supplanted modern dance techniques such as Graham, Humphrey-Limon, and Cunningham, and it also frequently serves as an effective complement to other techniques that dancers may acquire, including ballet and hip-hop. Dancers trained exclusively in Somatics are also regularly seen on stages across the globe, and Somatics as an underlying influence on many different genres can now often be observed.

Given its pervasiveness and popularity, it is remarkable that so little scholarly attention has been paid to Somatics pedagogical philosophies and to its historical development. My former PhD student Doran George perceived this gap in the critical literature on dance, and specifically dance training, and wrote a dissertation tracing the development of Somatics that included an assessment of its ideological underpinnings. Prior to their untimely death, George had been revising the dissertation manuscript for publication as a book, and this edition reflects those efforts.

George was especially dedicated to examining the historical transformation of Somatics, a practice that in its early years had been largely implemented as an antidote to other dance techniques where dancers were incurring injuries. Particularly intrigued by the persistent appeal to the natural made by different generations of Somatics practitioners, George analyzed what a "natural way of moving" both enabled and repressed or excluded. They saw this critique as a way to enrich the practice and support its deeply valuable contributions to dance training and to understanding the body.

George's extensive transnational training and network of relationships with practitioners of various branches of Somatics provide an extraordinary window into this training practice and the artists and teachers who have specialized in and promoted it. Having studied Somatics in the United Kingdom, at the European Dance Development Center in the Netherlands, and at various schools and studios in the United States, George developed an intimate knowledge of the practices and forged strong alliances with many of its students and teachers. As a result, this book brings into the historical record many heretofore neglected artists and teachers, and it offers fascinating portraits of the daily lives and concerns of dancers.

The book also offers a cogent analysis of the ways in which training regimens can inculcate an embodied politics as they guide and shape the experience of bodily sensation, construct forms of reflexive evaluation of bodily action, and summon bodies into relationship with one another. George continually aligns the development of the practice of Somatics with social and political changes occurring in the various locales where it took hold, showing how it assisted in defining community and furthering its political as well as aesthetic goals. As such, George's research gives us a model for how to integrate the process of dance training into the body politic.

Throughout the editing process, I received support and guidance from Lionel Popkin, and I thank him heartily for his wit and generosity. I also thank Doran's mother, Ann Gilbert, and life partner, Barry Shils, for their support of this project. In attempting to find photos for the volume, I made contact with a number of Somatics practitioners, photographers, and archivists who have generously given their time in providing images and many helpful comments. In particular, I would like to thank Eva Karczag, Nancy Stark Smith, Jennifer Monson, Chris Crickmay, Graham Greene, Ros Warby, Nanette Hassall, and Dona Ann McAdams. In some cases, these exchanges also pointed toward different interpretations of the significance and reception of Somatics that, as the editor of another author's text, I did not feel I could respond to fully. I did endeavor to "fact-check" as best I could, and I apologize to those who might continue to feel misrepresented in this text. Nonetheless, I believe strongly in the value of this scholarly project, and I hope that it will provoke debate and significant further scholarly interest in this vital topic.

This book would never have come into being without the considerable efforts of a superb team of graduate research assistants: Arushi Singh, Ryan Rockmore, Jingqiu Guan, Barry Brannum, and Jacqueline Davis. I am immensely grateful to them and also to the two anonymous reviewers of the manuscript who gave detailed and very constructive comments. The folks at Oxford, and in particular Norm Hirshy, were a joy to work with, and I thank them for their support of this work.

Introduction

In Search of the Natural Body

Under the influence of regimens broadly known as "Somatics," late twentieth-century contemporary dancers revolutionized their training.[1] They instituted biological and mechanical constructs of the body as the guiding logic for dance classes, claiming to uncover a "natural" way of moving. In so doing, they drew upon early twentieth-century theories of postural and motional health, influenced by Darwinism and progressive education. Somatics used this conceit of naturalness to develop a new form of training designed to supersede Graham Technique and ballet training, which were thought to be harmful to the body because of their demand to fulfill specific aesthetic ideals.[2] Convinced of the importance of Somatics, practitioners initially worked with meager resources and through small, alternative venues and institutions, forging transnational alliances of pedagogies and aesthetics in the United States, Britain, The Netherlands, and Australia, among other locales. Yet by the end of the twentieth century, the training had found its way into many of the world's most venerable dance education programs, and choreographers who initially experimented with Somatics in a small community began to be featured in the transnational circuit of large concert houses.

This book chronicles a history of Somatics, examining how dancers conceived of and sourced nature and the natural to overhaul training, performance, and choreography beginning in the 1960s and continuing up to the end of the century. The ideological underpinnings of Somatics changed dramatically over this period, affecting studio procedures and the look and aptitudes of the dancing body along with creative and choreographic processes. Yet despite these changes, dancers remained consistent in the language with which they represented essential truths of the body that they claimed to access. Combining scientific metaphors with ideas from non-Western practices that they represented as ancient and mystical, practitioners believed they were retrieving lost corporeal capacities that were nevertheless still evident in children, animals, and supposedly primitive peoples.

The Natural Body in Somatics Dance Training. Doran George, Oxford University Press (2020). © Oxford University Press.
DOI: 10.1093/oso/9780197538739.001.0001.

Implementing this rhetoric, a community of practitioners had consolidated by the 1970s, proposing that their comprehensively inclusive concept of the body engendered an antihierarchical collective dance culture. Along with other subcultures of the era that turned to nature as a source of liberation, Somatics purported to resist outdated gender ideals and authoritarian training by finding personal authenticity in the body's fundamental motility. Yet, as I will argue, the centrality within the training of individual creative freedom, which fueled the rapid transnational uptake of Somatics, instantiated key principles of American postwar liberalism. Along with their American colleagues, British, Dutch, and Australian dancers believed that by displacing modern and classical aesthetics with natural anatomical functioning, they were reclaiming an inherent right to individual creative freedom.

By the 1980s artists had largely jettisoned the emphasis on collectivism, yet as they became entrepreneurs in line with the new economic culture of staunch individualism, the rhetoric about nature endured. Using signature choreography and emphasizing the uniqueness of different Somatics-informed pedagogies, they pursued careerism, all the while contesting a variety of conservative cultural agendas. By the close of the twentieth century, Somatics had achieved institutional status, embodying a new corporate ethics. The creative autonomy that dancers had won in previous decades now transformed through demands made upon artists in education and the professional field to prove that dance is constituted by boundless innovation despite the diminishing arts resources in an age of austerity. Throughout all these changes, Somatics continued to cultivate and promote the idea of a natural body as an invisible yet essential category of nature, one that, while appearing to be inclusive, nonetheless marked difference and enacted exclusion from its supposedly universal purview.[3]

While these are some of the conclusions I reached following my research on Somatics, my inquiry was initially fueled by a contradiction that I continue to ponder. On the one hand, Somatics initially promised to liberate dancers from oppressive training by being more respectful of the body and nurturing the creativity of each dancer. On the other, as I slowly came to realize, the Somatics education I received instituted conservative and exclusionary values. In the early 1990s I began study at the Dutch European Dance Development Center (EDDC) because the school's ethos matched my leftist convictions. The modern and classical approaches I witnessed in conservatories in my home country of Britain corresponded with a dictatorial culture precipitated by Thatcher's conservative government. Under the instruction of seemingly imperious teachers, students painstakingly repeated and perfected codified vocabularies of steps. By strong contrast, EDDC students seemed to research their own vocabularies based on an experiential understanding that they cultivated of anatomical functional imperatives. We believed we were working with culturally neutral "natural" kinetics that could engender artistic diversity, which I connected to values shaped by protesting against Thatcher's right-wing agenda. As an economically disadvantaged genderqueer young adult, I allied myself with various minorities, women, and the working class, all under attack in 1980s Britain. Moreover, by disbanding from codified vocabulary, disabled and nondisabled dancers invented new movement, involving wheelchairs, for example.

Yet this same education also largely excluded non-Western dance aesthetics and configured transgender expression as artificial. My effeminate movement and pronounced assibilation of words containing "s" sounds seemed not to be culturally neutral because they challenged prevailing beliefs about natural gender. So when I was told my voice was unnaturally high and was encouraged to work with male teachers to connect with my masculinity, I believed my femininity resulted from my bodily nature somehow having been thwarted. Southern European and non-Western students faced similar problems by coming from cultures that are represented as especially passionate, sexual, and mystical in Anglo, Germanic, and Nordic contexts. Like me, these students found that the school's dominant aesthetics marked them as nonnatural. Thus, despite its progressive intentions, the EDDC stratified bodies as being more or less authentically connected with nature, and although I (and others) questioned the pedagogy's premise of neutrality, it was difficult to challenge because it was bolstered by generally accepted scientific metaphors.

To reveal distinct cultural values that Somatics embedded in the concept of nature, this study compares significantly different ways in which Somatics has been implemented over time in different locations. Distinct political, economic, and social factors affected Somatics practice, which resulted in contestations within each of its communities. However, dancers framed their disagreement through the discourse that movement's physical principles that were inherent in the body were being discovered through various implementations of the training. In this way they resolved the conflict between the idea that they were accessing natural movement while at the same time cultivating diverse practices, based on the assumption that their experimentation gave rise to different possibilities.

To the degree that all practitioners invested in the regenerative potential of nature, they shared in dubious perspectives about cultural difference. Most practitioners claimed to heal the body by looking beyond the "modern West" to a largely undifferentiated ancient Orient, and inward to a lost, timeless, savage nobility still evident in children, animals, and vaguely defined primitive societies. The ubiquity of naturalness overshadowed the political significance of such representations, erasing cultural differences and historical specificity.[4] As I will discuss in chapter 1, practitioners swept away the memory of racist and eugenic rhetoric in early twentieth-century Somatics as if it were irrelevant to more enduring insights. They established unimpeachable bodily truth by virtue of its discovery in such distinct contexts as Zen Buddhism and martial arts, which each supposedly exhibited truths similar to Western physiology and evolutionary theory. In so doing, they felt they had recuperated a body from various traditions that provided comprehensive inclusivity. As the twentieth century progressed, artists contested the conceit of universality by emphasizing cultural difference. Yet by the new millennium, Somatics still manifested a canonical universal body as an ostensibly invisible category of nature that purported to account for human ontology even while it marked difference and enacted myriad exclusions from its supposedly universal purview.

In my research, I put to use an internal conflict in which I simultaneously identify with and reject Somatics. This arose because I grew as an artist through changes in my physicality and values as I embodied the training, even though the conceit of naturalness was oppressive. My experience in the studio, and the broader culture of which the EDDC was a part, has afforded me detailed insight into the meanings with which the training and choreography are infused. In the eighteen years since my graduation from the EDDC, I have continued to use Somatics as a dancer, choreographer, and teacher, and over the course of that time I have remained in contact with my teachers as well as forged connections with other artists working with the training. This has allowed me a greater appreciation of how physical aptitudes are cultivated in classes and represented in concert dances, all of which embody Somatics-related values. I have attuned myself to how the physical experiences and choreographic strategies associated with Somatics translate into the aesthetic and ideological convictions that form artistic and social identities.

This study therefore builds on questions I asked about the assumptions of the culture in which I participated. In this sense, I follow Cynthia Novack's method in *Sharing the Dance: Contact Improvisation and American Culture.* As a participant-observer, she analyzes a community that grew up around Contact Improvisation (CI) by ricocheting between distance and proximity to that culture. In a similar manner, I interrogate the aesthetics and ideology that are produced in Somatics classes, and that are evident in concerts. To verify my interpretations, I collected teachers' and students' written and spoken views on different methods, the labor they entail, the associated aesthetic effects, and the perceived benefits of Somatics. In addition to the use of participant observation and oral history, I have drawn on publications that address the development of the field as reference materials. Beginning in the 1970s, dancers formed *Contact Quarterly* (CQ) and the *Movement Research Performance Journal* (MRPJ) in America, as well as the British *New Dance Magazine* (NDM) and the Australian *Writings on Dance*, which all had various regional, national, and transnational circulations. Along with other press, institutional and personal archives, articles, letters, reviews of concerts, and interviews, the journals document debate and commentary, offering insight into the range of perspectives about Somatics. These documents enhanced my understanding of how practitioners interpreted and applied Somatics ideas.

The Somatics network grew, in large part, because artists believed not only in the power of the regimens to train the body but also in their potential to fuel new choreography. Because dance establishes values in a symbolic exchange between performers and audiences that both confirms and diverges from artists' own understandings of their work, I have endeavored to identify these values as, in part, reflections of the various conditions, political and economic, as well as aesthetic, that impacted the way dancers were working. As I will show, these influences extended beyond the studio and the concert stage into the organizations and other activities through which artists developed and sustained their community. The considerable differences in the distinct historical and geographical communities, therefore, showed up in dance classes and company structures, venues, publications, institutions, and the dancing bodies themselves. To establish some sense of cohesion within such a dynamic and diverse community, I read the regimens as cultivating comparable physicalities that achieve contrasting meaning in different contexts, and I also identify differences in the way that artists choreographed common beliefs in Somatics about the nature of the body.

Explanations that configure the significance of the body as beyond culture, such as those proffered by Somatics, forfeit an understanding of how social forces are embodied through dance. To reveal the meaning that dancers construct through the idea of natural bodily capacity, I therefore position my research alongside dance scholarship that analyzes the symbolic significance of corporeality and its motion. Like many dance practitioners, some scholarly approaches insist that the value of Somatics lies precisely in its ability to connect dancers with precultural bodily dimensions and in so doing reinforce a commitment to "foundational" aspects of the body that contribute exceptional understanding to the humanities. I argue, however, that this eclipses the potential for a greater appreciation that comes from theorizing movement as a cultural site of meaning making. To challenge the exclusion and marginalization in which Somatics participates, scholarship needs to account for the cultural biases embodied through and produced by the training. This is particularly urgent now that the regimens are so widely used in dance education.

Dancers have often bolstered the universality of their capacities, like kinesthetic awareness, by projecting specificity, or that which appears to be culturally conspicuous and nonneutral, onto nonwhite and non-Western bodies. In many cases, they inherited this strategy from modern dance. Even as dancers rejected modernist master narratives by using the Somatics idea of nature, they formulated a concept of neutrality similar to that established by previous generations of white artists. In this sense, I position the regimens within an aesthetic tradition that Susan Manning identifies in *Modern Dance Negro Dance: Race in Motion*, where she exposes the previously uninterrogated racial investments in the universality staged in American modern concert dance. I agree with Manning that it was against the racialization of African American bodies that white dancers seemed to transcend cultural specificity, an insight I also bring to the role of Orientalism. Using research that celebrates modern and contemporary dancers' use of non-Western ideas, Somatics-based artists have projected cultural specificity onto the traditions from which they borrowed aesthetics and ideologies to achieve the universality of the body.

The projections in which Somatics participated, however, differed for bodies and practices associated with Africa compared with the East. I articulate this difference by building upon literature that aims to expose how racialization and whiteness work in dance through the construction of universality. Ananya Chatterjea, for example, delimits "postmodern" dance with the category "women of color" in *Butting Out: Reading Resistive Choreographies Through Works by Jawole Willa Jo Zollar and Chandralekha*. She argues that a white avant-garde configures African American and South Asian women as the custodians of history and culture to furnish themselves with access to the contemporary and the universal. Similarly, in *Digging the Africanist Presence in American Performance: Dance and Other Contexts*, Brenda Dixon Gottschild insists that postmodern dance erases the influence of black culture. Extending this argument to Somatics, I argue that the practices—in the process of claiming to "peel away" cultural imposition and "reveal" precultural aptitudes, many of which exhibit what Gottschild calls Africanist aesthetics— end up erasing the influence of black culture.[5] Informed by Chatterjea's and Dixon Gottschild's combined frameworks, I remain attuned to how the regimens participate in the appropriation of traditions represented as Eastern, while erasing the influence of African traditions. At the same time, they mark and thus risk the exclusion of non-Western bodies and nonwhite bodies.

We gain greater appreciation of the political contradictions in artists' practice through a nuanced understanding of how dancers construct a naturalized idea of the body and how artists use the concepts they have at hand to negotiate their historical exigencies. For example, Gay Morris elucidates the circumstances that shape discrepancies in the significance of Merce Cunningham's midcentury dances. Morris addresses the contradiction at the heart of my subject, because, while she argues that Cunningham resisted textual meaning through evocation of a seemingly universal body, she sees that the strategy was socially specific. Staging dance as meaning nothing more than corporeal movement, and therefore culturally neutral, seems to exhibit the potential of the body to contribute meaning not produced elsewhere. Yet, Morris clarifies that Cunningham addressed specific social circumstances and that his strategy cannot be universalized.[6] She points out that in the 1950s and 1960s his approach only worked for white artists because of the way black artists were marked in modern dance, and she characterizes his approach as representing the flux of nature, for which he drew on Zen ideas. Like Morris, I identify the cultural labor in which Somatics practitioners engaged through their processes and beliefs, as well as the conditions that shaped their interventions. As they resisted obvious meaning, Somatics practitioners often disbanded polarized gender ideals still evident in classical and modern aesthetics, but they continued to marginalize nonwhite bodies, among others.

Thus, this project identifies the meaning making in dance, as it is intertwined with social circumstances, by building on scholarship that interrogates bodily kinetics and experiences as a means of constructing culture.[7] Rather than situating the origin of meaning in a body to which language is external, or in a mind distinct from the body, I construct Somatics as a "movement culture" in which textual and physical significance are enmeshed along with dancers' social circumstances. Therefore, this study builds not only on Novack's methodology but also on her argument that social arrangements are embedded in and extend from the dancing body. Not only do the dancers produce, sustain, and transfer their values in and through the sensuous and physical dimensions of kinetic experiences, but also the patterns of social organization extend from and support the meaning constructed in the dancing. Economic and other social circumstances condition bodily significance, influencing dancers as they make sense of, and reach for, practices of living based on beliefs they cultivate in their dancing. Movement culture, then, represents a nexus of influences that cohere around a dance form. Yet the members of the community consciously draw upon some of them while denying or being unaware of others.

The complex nature of my subject has required a combination of ethnographic and semiotic analysis in which I establish tropes that underpin dynamic community values that simultaneously embody the broader social meaning through which corporeality is constructed. Defining a discursive field necessitates a level of abstraction in which, as Novack puts it, "exceptions, contents, and nuances disappear in favor of generic characterization and hyperbolic categorization."[8] With the caution that she brings to identifying the values embedded in a dance practice, Novack models how to apprehend the nuances that give shared values meaning. She insists on applying her insights to "a multiplicity of ethnographic realities [that] shape the unique and historical occasion of any dance," and therefore questions "the transmission and transformation of dance from one cultural setting to another, as well as from one historical period to another."[9] By moving between abstraction and specificity, she reveals meaningful change in CI, and I follow her approach to reveal comparable distinct uses of Somatics.[10]

By articulating community values in and subject to changing circumstances, I also build upon scholarship that traces rapid change in late twentieth-century dance. For example, Emilyn Claid, in *Yes, No, Maybe . . . Seductive Ambiguity in Contemporary Dance,* chronicles dancers' rejection, in the 1970s, and re-engagement, in the 1990s, of theatrical display. Claid contrasts the changes in artistic values introduced, in part, through Somatics with an intransigent "theatrical economy" that demands the artists seduce their audience, and this elucidates how broader political questions interface with dance through ideology that is specific to the art from. The community of artists upon whom she focuses overlaps with my subject. To build upon her insights, I analyze the aesthetic developments as affecting, and as intertwined with, shifts in the social field in which they occur. Somatics develops alongside changes in educational institutions and concert houses as part of a dynamic social field.

Tracing the broader sociohistorical processes in which dance is embroiled helps to account for the conundrum in which Somatics exhibits substantial variance while sustaining a consistent theory of the body. As referred to earlier, the regimens extend a mid-twentieth-century liberal ideal of universal individual freedom through the diversity with which artists implement a theory of the natural body. This thesis depends on analyzing the art form and bodily significance within broader social change. In this sense my project applies to Somatics an art historical framework developed by Serge Gilbaut in *How New York Stole the Idea of Modern Art: Abstract Expressionism, Freedom, and the Cold War*. He links the global success of American painting to the post–World War II ascension of liberalism, thereby departing from the tendency in his field to treat aesthetics independently from social change. Adapting Gilbaut's lens, I draw on theories that align cultural change with economic development; scholars have shown that the arrangement and categorization of working practices entail symbolic schema that affect how people see themselves.[11] Translating this argument to dance, I argue that Somatics rhetoric has manifested the idealization of universal individual freedom exhibited in both postwar American foreign policy and the late twentieth-century economic cultures that emerged in the Western hubs I address.

By insisting that the contextual conditions in which Somatics develops are integral to the body that dancers construct, my project differs from most writing on the subject. Commentators largely tell the story of a particular pioneer and/or the regimen in recognition of what has been achieved,[12] or they explain how Somatics processes work to promote the value of the regimens for dance education.[13] In all these cases, by accepting the basic presumptions of Somatics, writers conceal the cultural labor of the artists they address. In contrast with these approaches, I have attempted to recognize what artists achieve by conceiving of the body as natural or beyond textual meaning, and yet I contest their belief that they are uniquely accessing natural capacity in their dancing, and thereby reveal some of the cultural biases that are obscured within the rhetoric.

Each of the three chapters that make up this study traces a different dimension of the history of the development of Somatics in relation to political, cultural, and aesthetic contexts. Despite the fact that enormous uniformity in the conception and philosophy of the body went largely unchallenged, training and concert dance in different decades manifested and produced significantly different meanings. Between the 1960s and the end of the twentieth century, the dominant values within the community using Somatics transitioned from emphasizing collective spirit to individual self-representation and, ultimately, began to embody workforce compliance, all of which depended on the development of a transnational community of practitioners. Chapter 1 traces the development of Somatics as an approach to training as it began to develop in the United States at midcentury. Focusing first on the foundational teachings of F. M. Alexander, Margaret H'Doubler, and Mabel Elsworth Todd, I then examine the work of Joan Skinner, Bonnie Bainbridge Cohen, Susan Klein, Elaine Summers, and others to show how these teachers and artists, as they overhauled the cultivation of dancing bodies through the regimens, established a confluence between individuality and universality. In oppositional response to protocols that were institutionalized in modern dance, these teachers sought autonomy over their bodies and individual creative freedom. They claimed that by recovering universal principles of human movement, they could achieve bodily authenticity and thereby resist aesthetic imposition. To conceive of a transhistorical and precultural body, they constructed a lineage that consolidated Progressive Era and midcentury ideals that they believed were the discovery of bodily truths. Focusing on texts and on studio-based directives and pedagogies, the chapter chronicles how the training continued to exhibit the confluence of individuality and universality, even as Somatics pedagogies and the contexts in which they were utilized transformed substantially. By focusing exclusively on the US context, I hope to show how the pedagogies were repeatedly rejuvenated by generations of practitioners through recourse to an overriding discourse governed by the logic of the natural.

Chapter 2 then examines the transnational dissemination of Somatics training, returning to the 1970s and 1980s to show how the pedagogies began to be exported. Practically and ideologically underpinned by postwar American expansionism, Somatics pedagogies initially rode upon the coattails of the earlier American export of modern dance. In this sense we see how, in its confluence of individuality and universality, the training embodied the liberal ideals of the US expansionist project. Artists disseminated Somatics as a set of universal bodily truths accessed through the regimens that would provide a foundation for individual creative freedom. By instituting the regimens in various regional and national contexts, they verified the universality of Somatics. At the same time the American origins of liberal ideals disappeared because dancers developed unique local approaches as they tackled distinct conditions and even critiqued some tendencies in Somatics that were associated with American cultural dominance. Artists also patched together transnational support at a time when establishments were hostile to Somatics, so their liberalism seemed independent of transnational flows of culture through powerful institutions. Meanwhile, an essentialized natural corporeality proved its use in galvanizing creative freedom as the synthesis of locally specific Somatics bodies that were interconnected by a transnational discourse of geographical significance. New York established a professional and innovative Somatics body at the network center; a Somatics body of respite emerged in New England, one that escaped New York commercialism; British dancers constructed a Somatics body of political and social significance against what they saw as apolitical American dance; Dutch educators synthesized a Somatics body in flux, resisting a relationship to any single dance context; and Australian dancers asserted a Somatics body as a new frontier in a postcolonial cultural independence movement. The process of transnational expansion established the veracity of Somatics universality, yet dancers also asserted individual creative freedom as central to the training because they contested the disapproval with which they were met by local modern dance establishments.

Chapter 3 then analyzes the concert-stage choreography produced with Somatics-trained bodies and ideas, focusing specifically on its development in New York City. Based on the theory that the natural body brings together individuality and universality, choreographers represented postwar liberal ideals through the way they framed the dancers' identity in the artistic process. Concert dance fueled the interest in Somatics because artists argued that the training liberated the dancer from the authoritarian grasp of ballet and modern dance, producing new possibilities for choreography. I return to the three phases of development in training identified in chapter 1 and analyze three corresponding approaches to choreographic strategy defined by distinct dancer-choreographer relationships. These exhibit change over time as well as some regional variations. The first strategy, "processing," exemplifies antihierarchical collectivism because artists first developed the approach to collapse choreographic authority into the dancers' experiences of moving based on natural functional imperatives. A second strategy, "inventing," drew from the Somatics body new vocabulary with which choreographers established an individual artistic signature. They did this by collaborating with Somatics-trained dancers who contributed creative autonomy to the making of dance. A third strategy, "displaying," restored the choreographer's authority but still extended liberal ideals by staging "newly liberated subjects." This third approach emphasized the choreographer's signature as an artist, which manifested in valuing dancers for the appearance of the movement they performed. Because this approach recapitulates the ideas in modern and classical dance that Somatics initially rejected, the strategy represents the cessation of an experimental community.

I begin the book by looking at training to emphasize the role that constructing bodies in the studio plays in the formation of contemporary dance culture. The second chapter focusing on the dissemination of Somatics is intended to emphasize how the character of a technique is specific to the circumstances in which it is practiced. Yet, despite such specificity, my analysis reveals that American expansionism shapes the transnational context as an overarching ideology. Liberalism calls forth the local differences to verify its ideals. By articulating the temporal conditions that impact training in chapter 1 and the effect of geosocial dynamics in chapter 2, I provide a foundation for the analysis of representation in concerts in chapter 3. Throughout, I maintain a focus on the "natural," as a posture, a way of moving, and a way of being in the world, that enabled Somatics to both liberate and exclude, to encompass local and transnational social conditions, and to embed itself in movement and in artists' perceptions about aesthetic development.

1

Renewable Originality

Reaffirming the Natural Body throughout the Twentieth Century

As New York approached the end of the twentieth century, the front page of *Movement Research Performance Journal*, the premier publication for the dance community in which Somatics had been so central, declared:

> You can't fake release. You just copy what someone's body's doing when they're releasing and you can make your body look like that. The implications of that are that something will break down. . . . [I]t's not an evil thing—they're doing what their teacher's [*sic*] want them to do. They're reproducing. Dancers are trained to reproduce what they're seeing what is correct or desirable, but when it comes to release, that's one thing you can't fake. You can try but unless you're really releasing you're not releasing.[1]

In this claim for the exceptional status of release, Leslie Kaminoff references the deep-seated belief that Somatics, and specifically its practice of release, had revolutionized training. Kaminoff maintains that releasing cannot be copied because, along with the majority of her community, she believes in the training's ability to restore an innate natural capacity that other approaches bypass because they focus only on the way movement looks. Yet her focus on fakery also reveals that, by 1999, a style associated with Somatics that could be copied, called "release technique," had established prominence. This raised deep concern within her community. For four decades, dancers had believed that artistic authenticity, achieved by accessing the natural body, had protected them from pollution by institutional and commercial forces. Kaminoff's sentiment exemplifies a broader desire to protect the value of Somatics against what the community saw as the institutionalized pedagogies in modern dance and ballet, regimens that emphasized copying and perfecting specific movement patterns. Rejection of these training regimens underpinned the justification for Somatics and informed the choreography that its practitioners created.

The Natural Body in Somatics Dance Training. Doran George, Oxford University Press (2020). © Oxford University Press.
DOI: 10.1093/oso/9780197538739.001.0001.

Despite Kaminoff's belief in the natural foundations of the training, this chapter reveals how Somatics, although certainly marginal to other approaches for most of the late twentieth century, had always embodied specific styles. I hope to show that beginning in the 1960s, artists constructed a narrative of the lineage for their pedagogy that reached back to the early twentieth century. Building on early texts on bodily health and their attendant practices, artists at midcentury focused on the concept of nature that the earlier pioneers had developed with its implications for a natural posture and motion. Whereas the earlier texts contained within them certain assumptions about racial, cultural, and class categories that determined who could benefit from natural capacity, artists in the 1960s accorded natural capacity to every body. Nature thus achieved a new inclusivity at midcentury as dancers shifted the body's essence from being defined by aggregate social categories to one that was individual and universal. By emphasizing scientific rhetoric in the regimens, midcentury dancers focused on what they saw as precultural bodily dimensions, thereby divesting the training of troubling social and evolutionary theory. Moreover, based on their understanding of Eastern ideas, they validated receptivity to nature as a critique of the Western ego, a new orientation that empowered individual dancers as they struggled to overcome authoritarian dimensions of culture. Later generations of Somatics practitioners perpetuated the naturalization of individual receptivity, thereby continuing to universalize early twentieth-century ideas, establishing a prediscursive and transcendent corporeality as a source of inspiration and as a form of critical response to other training regimens.

In what follows, I focus on three distinct reconstructions of nature undertaken within US-based Somatics that reinvented its universal principles and their capacity to manifest individually. These shifts occurred between the 1960s and the end of the twentieth century. Prior to that I examine some of the early and midcentury epistemological foundations that established key ideas as touchstones to which dancers returned again and again. These foundations, based in early twentieth-century ideologies with their racial, cultural, and class prejudices, profoundly influenced Somatics, even though midcentury theories attempted to endow Somatics with a newly minted conception of the natural body as both universal and individual.

To trace these changes in Somatics training, and the impact on its community of practitioners, I analyze how the studio procedures, through which dancers felt they accessed nature, transformed to respond to the artistic challenges that arose in different decades. By examining the historical development of Somatics and its correlation with broader social issues, a process of sedimentation is revealed in which certain principles withstand the transitions in the training and thereby achieve natural status. At the same time, it becomes possible to track how the regimens themselves are not stable sets of ideas but instead develop their significance through the contexts in which they are used.

Early Twentieth-Century Somatics and Its Conceptions of Nature

To probe the ways in which the Somatics construction of a universally inclusive natural body originated in exclusionary theories, I first look at three Progressive Era educators whose ideas developed when nature was linked to social difference. Late twentieth-century practitioners reframed the ideas of F. M. Alexander, Margaret H'Doubler, and Mabel Elsworth Todd, who, beginning in the late nineteenth century, all participated in an American intellectual movement that explained racial, cultural, and class differences in evolutionary terms. Their theories emerged in the context of discourses that evaluated the proximity of different social groups to humanity's natural origins, and the value of such proximity for the process of civilization. Like late twentieth-century Somatics constructions of nature, the theories claimed to be universal, but rather than applying equally to all humans, they stratified social groups as either biologically distinct or having achieved a different level of evolutionary development. Within this historical context, Alexander, H'Doubler, and Todd theorized human physical form and function as related to learning and consciousness.

The training that Alexander developed was based in a prevailing distinction and stratification of the mind and body. Alexander insisted that by privileging intellectual over corporeal volition, the goal-oriented behavior in which Western epistemology was invested overrode natural physical capacity, which he argued is crucial to optimum functioning. For continuing human evolution, capacities intrinsic to the human body needed to be integrated with Enlightenment rationality; nature (the primitive) and reason (the civilized) needed to be conjoined.[2] Dancers were encouraged to reconceive the body-self in their training using his ideas. Specifically, Alexander argued that various "others" to a canonical white Western subject failed to embody "Man's Supreme Inheritance," the title of his first publication.[3] The fallen glory of ancient empires resulted from their failure to bring natural instincts under conscious control, according to Alexander, who thereby aligned his ideas with the logic used to justify colonial rule. At the same time, preindustrial agricultural workers living in Alexander's homeland demonstrated the loss

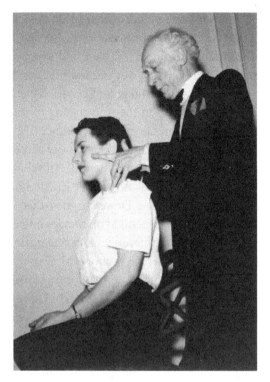

Figure 1.1. F. M. Alexander at work adjusting one of his patients (a journalist who interviewed him on occasion of his eightieth birthday) and encouraging awareness of certain muscles key to postural integrity.
Photograph by Australia News Information Bureau 1949. © The Society of Teachers of the Alexander Technique Archives, UK.

of mental capacity that results from reverting to nature.[4] He further argued that Africans could be approximated to animals that rely on base instincts, suggesting that their physical evolution extended beyond their mental capacity and lack of moral consciousness.[5] Civilization could supposedly only avoid the debauchery of antiquated empires, avert lower-class ignorance, advance above inferior races, and access its supreme inheritance through a new bodily consciousness to which posture training was integral.

Alexander ultimately ceased to stratify human groups in his theory of advancement, which probably reflects changing social mores and the mutually influencing intellectual relationship he enjoyed with progressive education pioneer John Dewey.[6] However, to grasp the cultural work that the technique does, we must appreciate its dependence on Progressive Era ideas about the "primitive" and "civilized" mind. The construction of nature through social categories, which later practitioners erased with an individualized postrace, postclass concept, remains embedded in ideas that Alexander shared with Dewey. Opposed to conservative interpretations of evolutionary theory that proposed innate limitations of the primitive mind as an explanation of economic and other disadvantages, Dewey argued that social ills like poverty could be solved with pedagogy that integrated Darwin's insights about natural development.[7] Dewey insisted upon the universality of intellectual capacity and the role of the social environment in its development.[8] Every human being could expand beyond the primitive mind, but Dewey agreed with Alexander that the body represented a crucial component of consciousness and, hence, of that process. In the same way that Alexander insisted on the importance of connecting with motor capacities, Dewey argued that intellectual development and social advancement depended on marshaling essential primitive capabilities.[9] He explained social differences as a linear progression between primitive and advanced cultures, which mirrored the evolution of the species, but accorded all human beings equal potential for improvement.[10] Although intrinsic to everyone, the primitive mind, which Dewey and Alexander agreed must be utilized in education, nonetheless accrued its definition from the kinds of distinctions between social groups articulated in *Man's Supreme Inheritance*.

Michael Gelb's *Body Learning: An Introduction to the Alexander Technique* exemplifies the enduring impact of Alexander's theory of nature, and it remains a widely used text on Alexander's approach. Published in 1981, the book configures children, animals, and non-Western tribal people as unfettered by the culture that robs white Western adults of their natural physical capacity.[11] While he seems to resist biological racism by idealizing rather than denigrating Africans, Gelb locks noncanonical and non-Western bodies in nature (the primitive), where they either remain as romantic visions of the past or wait to evolve so that rationality and culture (the civilized) can be integrated. The way that Gelb reconfigures Alexander's work is instructive because it demonstrates how practitioners isolated the idea of physical principles from racial theory. Gelb attributes his understanding of the postural training technique to Alexander's work and even makes reference to *Man's Supreme Inheritance*, and he sustains the conceit that an understanding of evolutionary theory provides insight about the central role of posture in constructing consciousness. However, Alexander's participation in early twentieth-century racial theories is never mentioned.

Influenced by Alexander's theory of posture as a universal constant and potential for human salvation,[12] a second movement educator, H'Doubler, began to apply Dewey's and Alexander's ideas in a way that established a foothold for modern dance in the university in the 1920s. Her teaching profoundly impacted the development of dance education generally and Somatics specifically.[13] She critiqued mind-body dualism by insisting that physical movement promotes learning, and thereby established the primitive mind as crucial to the intellectual, moral, and spiritual development of women.[14] To this end, her methods emphasized investigation and experience, encouraging students to investigate their own bodies through touch and to work together

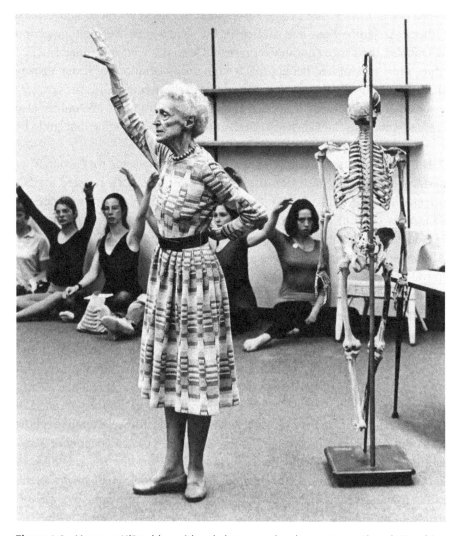

Figure 1.2. Margaret H'Doubler, with a skeleton nearby, demonstrates the relationship of scapula to humerus by holding up her arm in a gesture that is imitated by her students seated on the floor. Mills College, Oakland, California, 1972.
Photograph by James Graham. Courtesy of UW-Madison Archives.

and reflect on their findings. For example, to feel and reflect upon organic functional motion, H'Doubler's students took turns testing the range of motion of one another's joints while relaxed.[15] They also explored joint movement and crawled to sense shifting weight transference in their bodies. It is these methods that show up in late twentieth-century Somatics as the exploration of culturally neutral, essential kinetic principles. H'Doubler, however, working in the early twentieth century, needed to recuperate movement from the lasting Victorian associations of the flesh with salaciousness,[16] and so she constructed a body that projected dubious morals onto raced and classed Others. As Janice Ross has shown, in her comprehensive monograph on H'Doubler, the dance educator represented jazz as "'wild' and 'unartistic.'"[17] Thus, she distinguished her approach from the associations of sexual display that attended working-class women dancing in theaters as well as the savagery associated with African American movement traditions.[18] H'Doubler also resisted public displays such as recitals and concerts of dancing that could be connected to inappropriate public displays for women.

H'Doubler focused on experience and process, displacing the "product" of performance, which undercut display, and, like Alexander, rejected a goal-oriented attitude, yet to engage the primitive mind as a way to navigate the dangerous cultural terrain for women of achieving bodily self-possession, H'Doubler stratified social groups much like Alexander and Dewey. As with Alexander Technique, H'Doubler's pedagogy seemed to lend itself to the removal of racist and class-superior projections, and her cultural agenda ultimately disappeared into scientific rhetoric. As a result, her middle-class, white students exceeded restrictive gender codes under the rubric of experiencing anatomy unencumbered by social mores. Similar to Alexander, H'Doubler distanced her approach from the racial and classed bodies that were tainted, and thereby reimagined the primitive mind as available for social development with respectability. To mid- and late twentieth-century dancers, H'Doubler's activities seemed to be focused on bodily realities rather than cultural differences.

The work of a third educator, Mabel Elsworth Todd, further exemplifies how mid- and late twentieth-century dancers established the independence of evolutionary ideas from social difference. In her 1937 text *The Thinking Body: A Study of the Balancing Forces of Dynamic Man*, Todd focused on phylogenetic rather than cultural specificity, articulating movement principles by differentiating human mechanics from those of other species. Her work, which became broadly known as Ideokinesis, functioned as a blueprint for Somatics exploration of the body.[19] Yet, even though she refrained from social differentiation like that of Alexander and H'Doubler, the primitive mind remained key to the benefits Todd attributed to her "Natural Postural Training." Like

Dewey, she universalized a human capacity for rational thinking, which she attributed to upright posture, in contrast with the unconsciousness she accrued to lower life forms.[20] Todd also affirmed the crucial role of the primitive mind in social development, even though she refrained from defining it in terms of distinct social groups. She argued that functional efficiency depends on accessing the kinetic patterns of lower phylogenetic species that remain subconsciously locked in the human body as a remnant of evolution.

The similarities between Todd's, Alexander's, and H'Doubler's ideas made it possible for dancers, beginning in the 1960s, to synthesize their approaches in various forms of training.[21] H'Doubler and Todd both combined kinesiology, anatomy, evolutionary theory, and physics, and Todd's students also engaged in inquiry through physical action and experience, which exhibited the idea of having "instincts" act upon an environment to emulate the evolutionary process. Like Alexander, Todd placed humanity at the apex of evolution by virtue of capacities afforded by upright posture as an indication of consciousness.[22] She also agreed with him that humans had yet to master upright posture, which they needed to do by incorporating the primitive mind. As a result, they would advance in moral, affective, and intellectual functioning.

Beginning in the 1960s, dancers related Todd's training to the conceptualization of consciousness in Alexander Technique and the use of anatomy in H'Doubler's pedagogy. Todd's use of science convinced them of the precultural status of the body she constructed.[23] By proposing that different species' anatomy is subject to and formed by principles of physics and mechanics, Todd seemed to reveal how bodily structure arises from organic necessities peculiar to the way an organism negotiates its environment.[24] She constructed human biped uniqueness against other endoskeleton organisms including fish, horses, and primates,[25] arguing that if students could marshal the efficiency with which their bodies were designed to meet environmental demands such as gravity, breathing, and being upright, they could achieve postural and motional hygiene.[26] With the maxim "form follows function," Todd theorized human kinetic specificity as an extracultural and universal truism from which optimum motion could be deduced.

Todd's approach to postural training was articulated through modalities in which students developed a kinesthetic map of anatomical function.[27] Like H'Doubler, she believed that she could train her students to sense the skeleton and its function, and thereby synthesize reasoned analysis with instinct, achieving advanced consciousness, again reflecting Alexander's ideas. For example, her students reduced muscular effort, thought to be excessive within a given activity, by focusing on images, which, while related to an understanding gained by studying diagrams and skeletons, were often poetic.[28]

Both Todd and H'Doubler integrated the primitive and civilized minds by teaching anatomical structure and function with the aim that students should feel, and feel in their bodies. By searching for solutions to natural limitations that were sensed in the body in relation to the environment, students were seen to emulate the evolutionary struggle.[29] They understood human kinetics as the experience of anatomical and environmental constraints on motion. Once again Todd used science to affirm the precultural nature of her images, arguing that neurological theory proved the effectiveness of the prompts.

Dancers applied the combination of ideas put forward by Alexander, H'Doubler, and Todd as if they were restoring a precultural psychophysical integration, by accessing anatomical structure and mechanics, with sensory exercises that combined rational capacity with inherent bodily knowledge. Yet the conceit that consciousness was benign and universal, and that the experience of anatomical knowledge was scientifically grounded, concealed how the pioneers had constructed lower and higher forms of action and sensation through values within a socio-symbolic field. Still, using the pioneers' ideas, later generations of practitioners argued that they could uncover a precultural corporeality. However, the terms "primitive" and "civilized" continued to impact Somatics throughout the rest of the twentieth century through the notion that anatomical structure affords intrinsic optimum capacity tied to elevated consciousness.

Midcentury Somatics and Its Construction of the Universal Individual

At midcentury, many dancers began to refashion consciousness as residing in an individual who achieves freedom from institutional constraints by connecting through the body to a new kind of universal cosmology. Although modern dance had recently achieved respectability and institutional validity for the first time, some dancers also began resisting what they viewed as the imposition of aesthetic standards and protocols that were instituted by the newly formed modern dance establishment.[30] Those who sought to challenge perceived constraints upon artistic freedom developed Somatics with the idea that each body-self was divesting itself of both external and internal authoritarianism. In New York, San Francisco, and Los Angeles, artists synthesized training and staged dance that they felt embraced corporeal dimensions being suffocated by aesthetic imposition. In so doing, they participated in a broader anxiety that individual freedom was under threat, which was a postwar response to fascist and communist totalitarianism, as well as the extreme government scrutiny led by Senator McCarthy.[31]

Those who were wary or resentful of modern dance's institutionalization developed alternative cosmologies as a foundation for consciousness
by synthesizing early Somatics with what they saw as Eastern ideas. They
thought that the imposition of early modern dance severed the mind from
the body in a peculiarly Western fashion, and therefore set about revising
early twentieth-century Somatics. In contrast with Judeo-Christian
traditions, various Eastern philosophies seemed to facilitate the integration of creative resources found in corporeal nature and not graspable by
consciousness. Although "establishment choreographers" such as Doris
Humphrey had in fact drawn upon Todd's work, and in turn influenced
Jose Limón,[32] and Ruth St. Denis, Ted Shawn, and Martha Graham liberally borrowed from Eastern cultures, midcentury dancers believed they
were working with a new epistemology that was distinct from any already
integrated into modern dance. Drawing eclectically from yoga, Zen meditation, Tai Chi, and other martial arts as well as Buddhist and Confucian
philosophies, they constructed practices that did not necessarily resemble
these pursuits, as St. Denis and Shawn had done, but instead informed the
core values.

Eric Hawkins and Merce Cunningham pioneered in establishing key
Eastern philosophical ideas from which Somatics could borrow. Hawkins
pioneered training that purportedly engaged nature's indeterminacy,[33] while
Cunningham challenged institutional protocols by proposing that dance is
about nothing other than human movement for which anybody can be an aesthetic conveyer.[34] Hawkins sought "human movement, when it obeys the nature of its functioning, when it is not distorted by erroneous concepts of the
mind."[35] His manifesto exhibits his application of Todd's insights, which he
understood to prove scientifically the Zen concept of "receptive mind." Along
with opposing the use of physical force, Hawkins also valued indeterminacy
and immediacy. His training rejected the predetermined outcomes that his
milieu began to associate with established modern dance. Ideas like those
pioneered by H'Doubler, therefore, reissued through Hawkins's work where
his focus on kinesthesia in the idea of "Think-Feel" emphasized how voluntary control could be surrendered to bodily logic to achieve greater ease.[36]
By working with Todd's students Barbara Clark and André Bernard, Hawkins
and his dancers felt they unlearned habits accumulated in Graham and classical trainings.[37] The use of muscular force therefore became associated with
a willful Western ego compared with the lower muscle tone suggested by
Zen.[38] Cunningham contributed to this viewpoint by arguing that his Zen-
influenced aleatory composition was receptive to the nature of moving bodies
in time and space.[39]

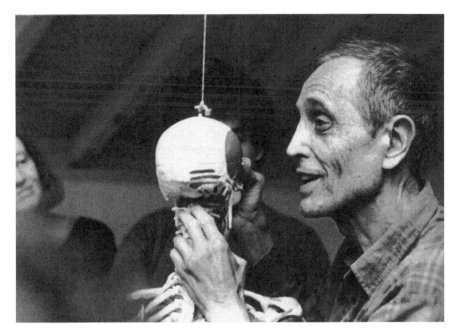

Figure 1.3. André Bernard teaching how to soften and deepen "the pit of the neck" in the area of the base of the skull at a workshop called "A Creative Approach to Human Movement and Body Alignment" organized by Ursula Stricker in Bern, Switzerland, sometime between 1991 and 2000.
Photograph by Hugo Lörtscher.

In contrast to Graham, who increasingly acquired the reputation of instructing the body to serve a willful expressive intent, Hawkins's and Cunningham's receptivity to nature emerged as oppositional to her perceived authoritarianism.[40] Some dancers saw her technique as artificial because they saw the use of force in her training as singularly directed toward achieving virtuoso display.[41] These dancers pursued alternative trainings, which they felt listened to the body and exhibited Eastern ideals.[42] Along with Hawkins, Allen Wayne taught classes emphasizing physical health by combining yoga and breath work with ballet and modern vocabulary done with reduced tension.[43] Dancers also perceived Alwin Nikolais's training as more humane and fulfilling of Eastern ideals.[44] In summary, midcentury modern dancers who rejected Graham technique sought physically softer approaches to care for their bodies by cultivating greater receptivity to nature through easing tension with lower muscle tone and focusing on anatomical structure and function.[45]

Despite the references to Eastern philosophy, in their own cosmologies, dancers configured the new training approaches as universal by displacing the context from which their ideas were drawn. For example, Cunningham's rhetoric suggested that his choreography reveals the essential thereness of movement, erasing the origins of the Zen ideas on which he drew while also proposing that he was exceeding the limits of Western epistemology.[46] The ease that Hawkins valued also appeared to be discovered in the body rather than cultivated, because the culturally remote philosophy of Zen and objective Western science appeared to be two contrasting lenses through which corporeal truth came into view.

Focused as they were on the midcentury rejection of Graham, artists lost sight of the fact that early modern dancers had long argued in favor of physical ease as providing access to more natural movement. Genevieve Stebbins, for example, had influenced Progressive Era artists with her interpretation of the training developed by French theater practitioner François Delsarte.[47] She connected relaxation and breath with inner emotion and external gesture in a theory of integrated body and mind similar to early Somatics.[48] Midcentury dancers cultivated ease in classes that built upon similar European theater traditions. They took "Sensory Awareness," pioneered by Charlotte Selver, and breath-based "Physical Reorientation," taught by Carola Speads, both of whom were indebted to Stebbins.[49] Also, Wayne had studied with Swiss movement theorist Émile Jacques-Dalcroze.[50] Ignoring or otherwise bypassing these genealogies that were associated with what they saw as artificial theatricality, dancers increasingly focused on the concept of natural ease. Not unlike the symbolic differentiation through the body that we saw with the terms "primitive" and "civilized," the new terms "force" and "ease," and "authoritarianism" and "receptivity" emerged as new socially indexed signs that were ultimately naturalized in Somatics constructions of the body.

Early on, New Yorkers largely modulated existing vocabulary with Somatics.[51] Hawkins, and teachers such as Merle Marsicano, as well as Nikolais's dancers, used Somatics in preparation for familiar exercises and phrase work, while Cunningham's approach was too balletic for some dancers seeking alternatives. Indeed, Novack points out "Cunningham did not practice 'all movement' even though he claimed that every movement could be dance, [and] Hawkins built his theatrical dance into . . . [an] immediately recognizable technique."[52] Meanwhile, the alignment and awareness classes taught by Speads, Selver, Clark, Bernard, and Lulu Sweigard, another of Todd's students, did not include dancing.[53]

By contrast, on the West Coast, Anna Halprin developed training and exploration that used Somatics to emphasize each dancer's uniqueness. Her approach seemed to fulfill the maxim that anybody could be an aesthetic conveyer. Like her New York contemporaries, Halprin actively rejected established modern dance, and although there was mutual respect among her and Hawkins, Cunningham, and Nikolais,[54] Halprin constructed her approach in opposition to the more refined appearance of their choreography.[55] With a similar agenda of renouncing imitation and display, Halprin reworked the pedagogy of her teacher H'Doubler to jettison the repetition of a pregiven form. Although the mid-1960s was the first time she was more than indirectly engaged with Zen, in the previous decade Halprin had already reframed H'Doubler's ideas as "presence in the moment."[56] She also recycled H'Doubler's concept of "synchronized awareness," the action of bringing together intellect, feelings, and motor response.[57] Her students explored moving while following kinesthetic physical impulses, all of which was framed in Eastern ideals popular among 1950s artists.[58] With her focus on individuality, Halprin aimed to replace exclusionary practice in established modern dance,

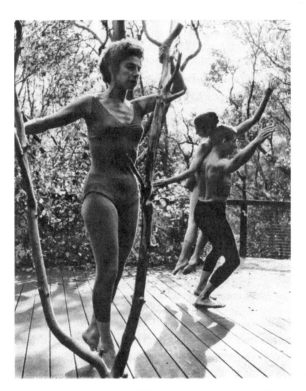

Figure 1.4. Anna Halprin, A. A. Leath, and Simone Forti in Halprin's *The Branch*, circa 1957, performed on Halprin's Dance Deck, Kentfield, CA.
Photograph by Warner Jepson.

which she had experienced, in part, based on her Jewish identity.[59] Appalled by institutional anti-Semitism in the 1930s, she subsequently redefined H'Doubler's pedagogy as inclusive, insisting that established modern dance was a tyranny in which the specific body of the choreographer was imposed upon every dancer.[60] Halprin combined H'Doubler's pedagogy with Bauhaus ideas about form and nature; she taught experiential anatomy through joint exploration, followed by the emulation of forms and movement in the natural environment.[61] Rather than practising an existing style, each dancer felt their movement was unique.

Like Halprin, Los Angeles–based Mary Starks Whitehouse aimed to recuperate individual creativity, arguing that established modern dance had forfeited this potential. Whitehouse, who danced for Mary Wigman and Graham, felt that by the 1950s, modern dance had robbed the body of its innate capacity for expression, replacing it with a stereotyped vision that manifested through an overinvestment in and institutionalization of virtuosity.[62] In her regimen, Authentic Movement, she aimed to reclaim dance from professionalism and restore it to humankind by releasing the private psychic process in Jungian-based dance therapy.[63] She insisted that, to fulfill their creative potential, practitioners must integrate all dimensions of the psyche through the body. Partaking in her decade's interest in Eastern philosophies, she argued that Zen and Taoist ideas can rebalance and thereby ameliorate the Western overvaluing of one side of various binaries.[64] Through the unification of opposites, individuals could purportedly move freely by simultaneously engaging as legitimate psychic components forces such as good and evil, spirit and body, masculinity and femininity. Whitehouse argued that an integrated psyche both was more akin to Eastern culture and represented the unification of East and West, facilitating the flow between individual, cultural, and primordial unconscious dimensions.[65]

Whitehouse constructed a body-psyche based on the primitive and civilized mind, pointing to "uncultivated" children's movement to demonstrate the free flow of energy. By contrast, she represented adult motion as that in which physical activity is reduced to necessary function. Like Dewey, she argued that Western society makes the civilized mind, from which the body is separated, the focus of learning. She protested, "We were, as little children, put at desks for hours at a time, increasingly, and told to keep still and learn."[66] In her rhetoric, the negative effect of social imposition creates inertia, while movement is synonymous with life. Furthermore, the primitive unconscious that resides in the body makes it impossible to lie despite one's intention to do so because even the physical tension produced by verbally expressing what contradicts one's true feelings is revealed corporeally. Whitehouse insisted: "The body is the physical aspect of personality, and movement is the personality made visible. The distortions, tensions, and restrictions are . . . [those of] the personality . . . the condition of the psyche."[67] Authentic Movement teaches that kinesthetic awareness enables the practitioner to discern between consciously arranged movement and the eruption of unconscious kinetic impulses. Practitioners aim to free the unconscious by abandoning concern about what looks attractive or how they think they should move, resulting in the application of Eastern knowledge to reintegrate body and mind, primitive and civilized.

Both Halprin and Whitehouse, like Hawkins and Cunningham, erased the cultural origins of their ideas by making contemporary innovation the purview of the West. Even though they all explicitly referenced Eastern philosophies, the specificity of the context disappeared because they represented the dancing as arising from precultural phenomena that were not indebted to Eastern movement traditions but were instead accessed through new interpretations of Eastern ideals. Along with Hawkins and Cunningham, Halprin and Whitehouse positioned the contemporary West as the site of rejuvenation for Eastern knowledge despite their criticism of Western epistemology. They stratified Western innovation over Eastern ideals by constructing the East as an original sight of integration to which they looked to develop procedures to access more natural and individual movement.

Thus, the biases and prejudices of early Somatics continued to haunt midcentury artists and educators, presenting problems for certain dance students. African American and Asian American dancers each faced distinct challenges from the largely white practice of Somatics. Both Gay Morris and Susan Manning have shown in their studies of midcentury dance how the modern dance establishment tended to represent black subjects as overly sexual and spectacular. Morris points out that Katherine Dunham's attempts to apply modernist principles to the study, translation, and choreographic deployment of "primitive ritual" was received by a white Protestant propriety as overly sexual and associated with commercialism. So despite Dunham's contention that the essence of the rituals was universal, the critical context within which her work acquired significance read the meaning as specific to the African body, which already symbolized sexuality and primitive physicality.[68] Manning shows how black dancers also contended with the status they had been given by the white critical establishment as having natural movement skill while also lacking the artistic distance necessary for modernism.[69] At the same time, Asian American dancers grappled with the implicit assumption that Eastern ideals, whose cultural specificity was now erased, informed Somatics approaches to movement exploration. For both groups, the concepts of nature, the primitive, and the universal were perhaps as much a burden as an asset.

In spite of these exclusions, the 1950s saw the stirrings of new techniques that synthesized Eastern ideals with early twentieth-century Somatics in opposition to modern dance's restrictive concept of the body, with practitioners of the new regimens often buttressing their arguments through narratives of recovery and healing.[70] In their explanations of Skinner Releasing Technique and Klein Technique, Joan Skinner and Susan Klein report gathering ideas in the 1950s to combat the effects of established trainings. In a related fashion, Bonnie Bainbridge Cohen argues she began seeing how institutional professional medicine stifled healing, which she then overcame with Body-Mind Centering (BMC).[71] These new pioneers insisted that a healthy dancer must be connected to a cosmological reality through their natural body. Their narratives sustained a tradition begun in the Progressive Era by Alexander, who in the rationale for his technique included the processes by which he healed himself from losing his voice.[72] Although Todd did not narrate her own story of healing, it does figure prominently in the teaching of her ideas.[73] Recovery, achieved by connecting with the new cosmologies, became a precultural mythical origin for Somatics.

As part of the focus on recovery, dancers believed that psychological and physical health are intertwined, a concept they also inherited from the early twentieth-century pioneers. Both Alexander and Todd distinguished their approaches from Progressive Era regimens that they felt did not address consciousness, and they configured the body as an independent arbiter of optimum psychophysical behavior with their claims to have discovered the futility of voluntarily instructing the body.[74] Alexander's story of the loss of his voice, for example, became a blueprint for the idea that the pursuit of preconceived goals interferes with intrinsic psychophysical connections. Cultural concerns seemed to be contrary to Somatics, because the regimens were accessing bodily propensities that were not available to consciousness. For dancers who were rejecting institutionalized aesthetics, the stories of recovery proved that more authoritarian training had interfered with bodily knowledge. Ease allowed psychological release and safeguarded health, while effort caused emotional repression and injury.[75] Dancers in the 1950s felt that through Somatics, they embodied authentic psychophysical processes rather than disciplining their bodies to artificially represent emotion.[76]

Displacing Aesthetics: Radical Inclusion in 1960s and 1970s Somatics

Throughout the 1960s, Klein and Elaine Summers developed Klein Technique and Kinetic Awareness, respectively, and Bainbridge Cohen created BMC, all in New York, while Skinner evolved her Skinner Releasing at the University of Illinois. Initially, all four approaches worked with known dance vocabularies but applied new sets of principles and new directives guiding the dancer's awareness to these vocabularies. Although Skinner eventually integrated exploration into her approach, she began by using Cunningham's lexicon.[77] Likewise, Bainbridge Cohen never saw her pedagogy as unconnected to various forms of dance technique. All four, however, sought more natural procedures to avoid injuries common in existing approaches and encouraged

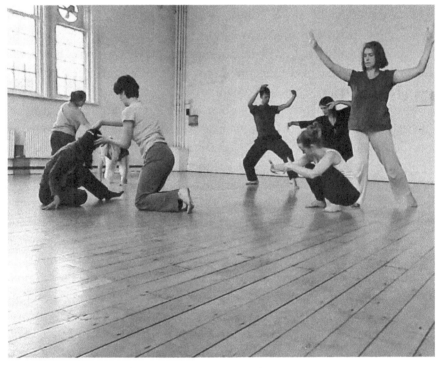

Figure 1.5. Members of the Skinner Release Network (SRN) dancing at an SRN Networking Day at the London Buddhist Arts Centre, September 8, 2013. From left to right: Sally E. Dean, Florence Peake, Ruth Gibson, Bettina Neuhaus, Alex Crowe, Polly Hudson, Maria Rita Salvi, and Gaby Agis.
Photograph by Rosemary Spencer.

their students to work reciprocally with the body at their own pace.[78] All four also professed the uniqueness of their approaches. By narrating personal recovery from modern dance injury in the explanation of their techniques, these educators established their credentials as commentators on and innovators in training. They also affirmed that, unlike early Somatics, they addressed the unique needs of dancers, while compounding the idea that Somatics was discovered in the process of the body's healing.[79]

In the late 1960s a group of Skinner's graduate students, Marsha Paludan, Mary Fulkerson, and John Rolland, along with Nancy Topf, who was a Cunningham guest teacher, consolidated an influential new regimen based on exploration by integrating their teachers' ideas with the kind of experimentation in which Judson choreographers had been engaged.[80] Anatomical Releasing established new studio procedures and a movement vocabulary that reflected new aesthetics that synthesized Todd and H'Doubler's ideas in classes very similar to early American dance education.[81] Following Todd's definition of bodily components such as bone versus muscle, and collections of joints, Anatomical Releasing students compartmentalized and then reintegrated the body to explore form and function in posture and motion.[82] Like H'Doubler's students, they explored knowledge of the skeleton close to the floor to reduce the challenges of gravity, while cultivating kinesthetic awareness of the minutia of change. Sensory images underpinned simple movement, followed by full body improvising.

Anatomical Releasing replaced theme, emotional expression, and virtuosity with the logic of working with intrinsic movement principles. Paludan, Fulkerson, Topf, and Rolland borrowed lying, sitting, crawling, and walking from Todd's work, which replaced Skinner's use of Cunningham's forms with vocabulary that was designated "pedestrian" as if it was natural to everyone.[83] By executing such simple action, students aimed to develop their awareness of their moving joints and the effects of gravity rather than practicing movement memory, balance, turning, and extension as they might in ballet or various modern dance techniques.[84] In this way, they sought to sense the mechanics of movement and also align themselves with Judson Church choreographers' focus on inclusion of pedestrian vocabularies.

Through the continuing development of both Skinner and Anatomical Releasing, along with BMC and Klein, 1970s Somatics reframed the midcentury rejection of modern dance by claiming to train dancers in a way that was unencumbered by aesthetics. Skinner recounts that while dancing for Cunningham, she discovered underlying natural forces that contrasted with the kind of volitional staging of a predetermined theme that defined her experience with Graham.[85] Exhibiting Alexander's and Todd's influences, she ultimately determined that instructing the body interrupts its unity with cosmological forces. As a result, Skinner Releasing ultimately jettisoned predetermined vocabulary altogether.[86] Meanwhile, Paludan, Fulkerson, Topf, and Rolland reframed H'Doubler's concerted rejection of spectacle,[87] while Summers and Klein established the independence of their approaches from aesthetics by virtue of body-based practices on which they drew beyond dance. In all the techniques, an emphasis on internal focus contrasted with the attention to the spectacular image of line, shape, and extension, visible in classical and increasingly modern dance studio mirrors. The process of refining the look of set movement made no sense in techniques that pursued indeterminate movement possibilities that would arise through connecting with the cosmos. Like 1960s task-based dances, 1970s Somatics insisted on the unintentional nature of the aesthetic effects of connecting with cosmic forces. Dancers followed sensation, believing that they were unifying body and mind, reframing Alexander's theory of consciousness as a means to escape from the visual focus of dance.

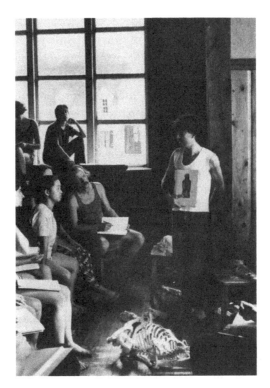

Figure 1.6. John Rolland with his students teaching an alignment class, Summer 1980. Photograph by Rebecca Lepkoff.

The use of "tactile feedback" enhanced dancers' convictions that they were escaping any concern with aesthetics. Touch in Somatics classes contrasted with how classical and modern teachers might give feedback using their hands. Instead of moving a student's body into the right form, Somatics teachers developed hands-on attention to help the receiver sense what was happening in the body while employing a particular image. The giver of hands-on feedback would not willfully move their partner, but rather invariably focus on the same image in their own and their partner's body, and imagine that they were breathing into their hands.[88] Beginning in the 1970s, pioneers and teachers of techniques increasingly offered individual sessions to dancers in which they used hands-on instruction, but Somatics classes also included the approach. Dancers often felt they became dramatically realigned or gained insight into habits through a hands-on approach.[89] In Alexander, Klein, BMC, and Todd's work, tactile feedback and associated verbal prompts had different names and subtleties.[90] In contrast with the other approaches, for example, Bainbridge Cohen included viscera with the skeleton, which I address in the following section, and Skinner designed "Partner Graphics," in which touch was often short and rapid rather than encouraging a slow contemplative engagement

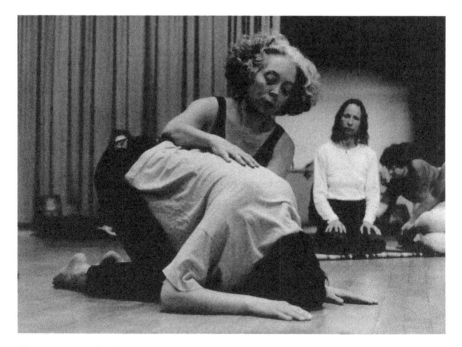

Figure 1.7. Bainbridge Cohen uses her "hands-on" technique to work with a student in 1995.
Photographer unknown. © Bonnie Bainbridge Cohen.

with sensation and image, as was often the case in the other techniques.[91] As a field of training developed, dancers also synthesized individual approaches to hands-on attention by combining ideas from the different regimens.

Despite the belief that dancers accessed indeterminate kinetic possibility by focusing on sensation, 1970s training exhibited recognizable vocabularies. Yet the forms were theorized as intrinsic to anatomical structure, and therefore "discovered" by dancers. Based on Todd's thesis that the most efficient movement surfaced earliest in the evolutionary process, students rolled and crawled on their bellies and all fours, gradually progressing toward walking on all fours and into biped motion. The new training therefore recycled early Somatics by redefining primitive movement as a source of capacity accessed through unconscious bodily response. This would help dancers avoid the injuries incurred in "overcivilized" classical and modern vocabularies.[92]

Skinner's and Bainbridge Cohen's 1970s pedagogies both vividly exemplify the idealization of experience thought to arise from unconscious bodily capacity. Skinner held that she discovered exercises by observing how students responded to her image work, which I analyze further in the next section.[93] Because dancers could not sustain her images while fulfilling specific movements, she discontinued teaching set material. Meanwhile, Bainbridge Cohen gathered ideas from her students, whom she saw as researchers of a body constantly changing and growing. Challenging medical authority as much as institutionalized modern dance, she configured the dancer's experience as empirical knowledge discovered in the process of following the unanticipated directions a body takes.[94] Educators instituted dramatic changes with the belief that only through direct responsiveness to the individual could the body's truth be uncovered.

A collaborative structure in Somatics classes further emphasized the necessity of hearing each dancer's experience to get at the truth of the body. For example, BMC and Anatomical Releasing students never stood in lines facing a teacher, but began in a circle discussing the function of a particular joint or organ, and then they usually dispersed around the studio to focus inward or toward each other and engage in sensing the bodily component with which the class began. Throughout or at the end of class, dancers often returned to a circle to share distinct experiences affirming their unique embodiment of nature.[95] Hands-on exercises convinced dancers that they were discovering bodily veracity because they were commonly surprised during the touch-based processes by the sensation of the location, size, weight, and dimensions of various bony or visceral components. Students often improvised individual spatial journeys in full-bodied dancing based on the more authentic bodily knowledge that they felt they had unearthed. Classes therefore claimed to both reveal the body that was masked in the artificiality of other training and validate the individuality that was repressed elsewhere.

Alongside Skinner, BMC, Anatomical Releasing, and other Somatics approaches, the duet form of Contact Improvisation (CI) began to develop in the early 1970s, and it similarly exemplified the idea of connecting dancers with primitive kinetic patterns to fuel endless movement possibility. Despite considerable disagreement among practitioners about the relationship between CI and Somatics, CI undeniably provided vocabulary and pedagogy for Somatics, while Anatomical Releasing and BMC, if not other Somatics approaches, were key to the development of CI.[96] Forms common in Somatics quickly became associated with CI, and this shared vocabulary was thought to be indeterminate and based on intrinsic principles rather than constituting a preexisting lexicon. As one of its main exponents, Steve Paxton wanted to eradicate decision making from dancing, and defined CI as following the moving weight exchanged in a duet.[97] Dancers experienced unpredictable changes in direction, speed, and action as they followed the shifting motion of their combined masses. Yet, to follow the collective moving weight of two people, each dancer connected their limbs, upper torso, and head to the momentum of their pelvis, the center of gravity. As in BMC and Anatomical Release, they used crawling, quadruped, and biped motion in which the pelvis can either lead or follow the limbs. CI and Somatics shared a class structure in which dancers pursued simple movement to sense their weight and bodily motion individually or in pairs, and then they improvised.

CI dancers also stratified movement along the Somatics spectrum of primitive and civilized through their warm-ups. Those that were trained in Somatics aimed to cultivate a responsive body, which Novack theorizes as central to the duet form.[98] Diane Madden recalls, for example, that Daniel Lepkoff, who introduced the form to many dancers who became key practitioners, often began with simple exercises working with touch and sensation to cultivate kinesthetic awareness. By developing facility in relative stillness that was then applied to larger movement, CI dancers invested in the idea that aptitudes, which contribute to the efficient execution of complex dancing, are more accessible in simple movement. They therefore reconstructed Todd's idea that kinetic patterns associated with lower life forms reside in the human subconscious while retaining her symbolic stratification. CI also shared with Anatomical Releasing metaphors from physics and mechanics, through which the movement vocabulary was constructed as foundational or primitive, in contrast with ballet's decorative and by consequence (over-) civilized lexicon. Dancers believed that through receptivity to terrestrial forces, they accessed kinetic efficiency in the combined mass of two moving bodies.

Lepkoff's approach contrasted with Paxton's, whom Novack describes as teaching the form in 1973 "largely by practicing it, with a few preparatory exercises."[99] Yet she also chronicles that most CI practice gradually integrated Somatics aptitudes.[100] Furthermore, Jowitt claims that as early as 1977, CI students learned BMC as part of the pedagogy.[101] Dancers aimed to feel gravity, friction, momentum, and the transmission of weight down the bones, which Paxton describes as "'reality' as transcribed by subjective experience."[102] This formulation echoes a comparable ideology in Somatics in which the dancer is thought to connect with intrinsic truths of the moving body.[103] He acknowledged that CI and Somatics shared principles even though he did not know the work when first developing the form.[104]

Somatics in the 1970s thereby reframed the use of science to claim the accuracy of its discoveries against prevailing concert dance aesthetics. Dancers believed that they brought objective truths to their art by mapping corporeality and its movement in a way that was detached from the emotional and sexual significance of the body. Anatomical Releasing relied on Clark's pared-down anatomical lexicon, while Klein claimed that practicing her exercises based on skeletal and muscular function promoted optimum biped capacity.[105] Although Alexander's and Todd's work influenced Skinner, she argued that scientific language excites the rational mind, inhibiting access to natural capacity. Yet she justified her poetic images using Sweigard's extension of Todd's neuromuscular control theory.[106] Also using neurological theory, Bainbridge Cohen reported that she had discovered that all the body systems generate "inner vitality," and that the outward expression of high "tone" in the organs and other bodily components promotes postural and motional hygiene, while a lack of vitality has the opposite effect.[107] Various clinical influences on Somatics also emphasized its scientific foundations.[108]

Convinced by the objectivity of their ideas, dancers believed that the regimens cut through the elitism they associated with modern and classical training. Somatics seemed to put information directly in the dancers' hands because many classes introduced models and diagrams from biology, physics, and mechanics to explain posture and motion. This felt more transparent than pedagogy based on a right or wrong way of executing a movement for which the teacher alone had the answer by virtue of being trained in the aesthetic tradition. Furthermore, Sweigard's student Irène Dowd used scientific rhetoric to argue that conventional training works against the body's natural tendencies, causing injury. She and Sweigard largely focused on training modern and classical dancers. Yet the Somatics community used Dowd's insights to bolster the idea that the kind of autonomy that dancers achieved in exploratory training helped them avoid injury.

Dancers' belief that they were working with natural movement principles underpinned their reframing of Somatics as direct democracy. David Held, for example, cites two principles that the 1970s training exhibited: decisions were in the hands of the people they concerned, and hierarchal governance was disbanded so as to dissolve conflicts of interest based on power differences.[109] Rather than being instituted as part of an imposed aesthetic, dancers believed natural forces shaped their movement choices. Yet they emphasized their individual experience of these shared bodily truths; and differences in the vocabulary they performed seemed not to be stratified, which affirmed dispersal of artistic authority. Novack identifies a confluence of individuality and universality in her account of how individuals experienced a group bond in CI.[110] Somatics similarly promoted unique journeys through a shared means, manner, and trajectory of development, and the studios had no mirrors in order to emphasize the focus on sensation.[111]

As radical and empowering as these resonances to democratic governance were, 1970s Somatics also consolidated several sets of exclusions, particularly through the use of science. The embodiment of scientific metaphors entailed orienting toward some bodily dimensions and away from others. Dancers were directed to perform as what Donna Haraway has termed "modest witnesses," de-emphasizing their sexuality and emotions, while focusing objectively on their bodies through the use of metaphors from science.[112] Somatics classes naturalized the performance of modesty because dancers believed that they were accessing intrinsic functioning rather than repudiating emotion and sexuality. For example, the Constructive Rest Position (CRP), which was central to both Alexander's and Todd's work, established itself as a staple of 1970s Somatics, and exemplifies how dancers cultivated propitious detachment. According to Alexander and Todd, the CRP demands the least effort to maintain skeletal alignment: with the body supine, the knees bent upward, and the feet flat on the floor, the head is placed on a book to position it effectively in relation to the neck and back. Dancers saw CRP as a way to establish a neutral sensory baseline by releasing excess tension and restoring functional kinesthesia from which they could sense and inhibit "unnatural" habits while moving to achieve what is known as the "natural" balancing reflex.[113] Reciprocal exercises like hands-on similarly engendered a chaste sensibility, because by focusing on anatomical ideas they wished to encourage in the receiver's body, both parties averted the emotional and sexual associations of physical intimacy. The kinetic ease that dancers achieved also seemed to verify the aim of functional efficiency, which affirmed a natural rather than cultural basis for the modesty.

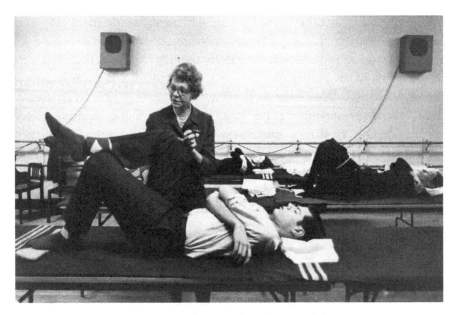

Figure 1.8. Lulu Sweigard assisting dance student Myron Nadel in an anatomy laboratory class at Juilliard, as all the students practice the Constructive Rest Position. April 1962.
Photograph by Susan Schiff for *Dance Magazine.* Courtesy of Juilliard Archives.

Somatics also cultivated detachment through the attitudes it fomented in dancers toward the body in motion. In the throes of sustained physical contact, for example, CI practitioners retained decency by emphasizing the mechanics of motion and averting erotic and emotional feelings. They accomplished seamless transitions by focusing on the action of bones relative to gravity and other forces. Meanwhile, under Alexander's influence, Skinner instructed her students to concentrate on the image to avert emotions that arose while dancing.[114] Dancers believed in the involuntary nature of the motility through which they performed such modesty, which further erased its cultural specificity. Skinner's students, for example, often reported being moved by images, confirming their pioneer's conviction that cosmic forces coursed through them. Recipients of hands-on also reported being moved without knowing how during their session, which they attributed to the activation of innate bodily processes.[115]

As much as the embodiment of scientific metaphors constructed a canonical body through the performance of modesty, the regimens compromised the access of noncanonical subjects to nature in various other ways. I have already pointed out how Gelb seemed to reverse Alexander's stratification of races and cultural groups while actually recapitulating his exclusionary conceit. Yet, by naturalizing pedestrian vocabulary, ease, and modesty, the seemingly new universal contemporary body of Somatics rendered the staging of black American traditions culturally conspicuous, and therefore outdated. At the same time, Brenda Dixon Gottschild argues that the influence of "Africanist Aesthetics" on what she calls postmodernism was erased. The belief that these skills were cultivated by connecting with natural capacity through scientific understanding obscured the impact of any cultural tradition.[116] Similarly, Somatics practitioners as modest scientific witnesses found in Eastern approaches ancient knowledge that could now be proven by science. The belief that the movement principles were transcultural bolstered the idea that they were unchanging and essential, even while the supposedly ancient insights were used to critique modern dance, which, in turn, erased the history of Orientalism.[117]

Paxton's use of Tai Chi exemplifies how dancers fused science with what they saw as ancient knowledge from the East. Due to the slow pace of the martial art, in contrast with the relative speed of modern dance, Paxton insisted he could track his reflexes as gravity acted through his anatomy. Using this knowledge, Paxton concluded that perception could be trained separate from action, and that dancers could be prepared for fast, disorienting movement in CI.[118] For example, an exercise called "the stand" aims to cultivate kinesthetic awareness of the reflexes that Paxton observed in Tai Chi: dancers sense subtle weight shifts, developing what he calls "a persistent delicate overall awareness of the reflexes which balance the body," which apparently "entrains" dancers to meet physical disorientation without panic.[119] Approaching Tai Chi as detached observer, Paxton extracted understanding of the body from it. By framing his insights within the discourse of Western science, the cultural origins and meaning of the martial art disappeared, becoming essential bodily truth recuperated for contemporary agency.

By the end of the 1970s, Somatics had established a new field of training built on ideas from the previous two decades. Sensing the radical democratic potential of the training, and largely oblivious to its exclusions, dancers and educators subsequently believed they were discovering and exploring intrinsic bodily structure and function rather than developing a style of movement. Although Somatics training diversified in the 1970s, dancers moved between different approaches that they saw as part of one big experiment. So, even though Klein, for example, worked quite differently from her contemporaries by insisting on the faithful repetition of specific actions to engage certain muscles, students saw her technique as part of the new field because it was couched in a similar rhetoric of restoring natural bodily capacity. Even though movement exploration was absent from her training, dancers believed they were working with the same bodily material, pursuing aims other than virtuoso facility directed toward display.[120] As we will see, the differences between these approaches became more important in the next two decades and beyond.

Individuality and Subjectivity in 1980s Somatics

Dancers in the 1980s sustained a lineage with 1970s Somatics while critiquing it in ways that dovetailed with the politics of the decade. A new generation, working alongside veterans, inherited a substantial discourse on the regimens grounded in the conviction that the dancer's identity and role in the artistic process could be reconceived with scientifically verifiable bodily knowledge that had been previously overlooked. Furthermore, the new dance culture that fostered these ideas asserted the foundational nature of its aesthetics. Two major trends emerged as the field diversified and grew. Some artists rejected collectivism to pursue career success with the new ideas, while others critiqued the conceit of universality, and the aesthetic of no aesthetics, even as they sustained collectivism. In both cases 1980s Somatics reconstructed nature to justify the new approaches that emerged.

Differentiation in the field benefited from new possibilities for the production and dissemination of choreography, as educators, programmers, and artists rode on broader economic changes. These developments, which I focus on in more detail in chapters 2 and 3, participated in the shifts associated with a political swing to the right among many Western governments. Most artists deplored the conservative cultural and economic agendas associated with Reagan in the United States and Thatcher in the United Kingdom, yet they adapted Somatics to capitalize on the new opportunities these administrations afforded. Even artists who resisted commercialization and conservatism often did so by foregrounding what they saw as staunchly individual rather than collective truths, which embodied the 1980s culture of self-interest, although with a critical agenda.

Already in the late 1970s new pedagogy emerged taking its logic from Somatics-informed choreography that was becoming increasingly visible. For example, through large theater engagements, Trisha Brown's work became emblematic of what could be achieved using Somatics.[121] She gained international status in the 1980s, and Somatics training was subsequently profoundly influenced by her work. Dancers wanted to learn the skills that they saw on large concert stages and in CI jams, so they flocked to classes based on the reproduction of hers and others' successful vocabulary, rather than finding their own movement responses. In a return to a 1950s model of Somatics classes, learning set phrases replaced individualized movement exploration. Although new classes based on set vocabulary were organized more like modern training, they distinguished themselves using the proposition that students were cultivating physical authenticity. For example, Lisa Kraus, who began dancing for Brown in the late 1970s, rejected what were seen as authoritarian teaching methods while offering training in virtuoso skills compared with Anatomical Releasing.[122] She taught the choreography she was performing, but Kraus gave her students the verbal prompts with which Brown developed her 1970s choreography as much as she demonstrated phrases. Based on her training in Todd's work and CI, she also encouraged her students to imagine the anatomical motion with which they were fulfilling the instructions.[123] Her emphasis on embodying movement principles framed the use of set kinetic forms in a way that was distinct from previous training models.[124]

Brown's 1980s company dancers followed in Kraus's footsteps. They prepared the students with exercises from regimens in which they were training, and then applied Somatics to the choreography they performed, using verbal prompts and hands-on.[125] Using images and instructions from regimens not designed for dance or in which dancing was not included, the teachers explained the dynamics of the vocabulary.[126] Vicky Shick applied a combination of approaches, while both Iréne Hultman and Shelley Senter focused on Alexander's work, and Diane Madden and Stephen Petronio emphasized the use of Klein Technique, as did Jeremy Nelson, who danced in Petronio's own company. Students faced the teacher and repeated phrases, but the classes began with contemplative internal focus, employing the logic that connecting with anatomical function and structure was essential to the execution of the set material. Rigorous self-awareness was seen as equally or more important than conventional skills like movement memory or mastering turns and balances.

Participants in these classes still understood them as vetoing the emulation of the look of dance because an authentic connection with the body was thought to underpin the motile efficiency that gave the vocabulary its artistic success. Using anatomical language rather than terms associated with classical training, teachers underplayed the technical demands of the vocabulary, and "getting the phrase" was represented as less important than focusing on one's own learning process. Shick, for example, rephrased passé from ballet as "lift the leg in parallel by softening the knee," which she believed changed students' execution.[127] Corrections took the form of anatomical instruction rather than reference to shape, and there continued to be a marked absence of mirrors in the studios. Set phrases therefore reinvented themselves as procedures to overcome habits, practice functional alignment, and develop motile efficiency. Like modern classes, the complexity of exercises gradually increased, yet students focused on sustaining kinesthetic awareness, and a class often returned to an anatomical insight set up in the beginning that informed the execution of a phrase.[128]

The use of Sweigard's CRP in classes exemplifies how dancers understood the difference between Somatics and modern, or classical, training. Prior to the class's beginning, dancers often practiced CRP rather than stretch, with the rationale that they were restoring a neutral sensory basis to avoid instructing the body. The CRP helped them to dive beneath the "habitual response" of goal-oriented behavior associated with skills developed in ballet and modern trainings. Furthermore, teachers used receptive-sounding terms like "allow" to describe how to embody movement, which they contrasted with terms like "gripping" or "pushing." It was not unusual to see students withdraw from phrases to practice CRP, which indicated that they were restoring a connection with unconscious capacity that had been lost in a goal-oriented drive toward executing a phrase.

The new pedagogy naturalized physical aptitudes that became identified with the material taught. For example, letting and flowing were powerful tropes in classes that became known as release technique. Dancers sequenced movement by reverberating a kinetic impulse outward from its center, controlling the direction and pace using kinesthetic awareness that they understood as the sensation of bony weight producing muscular ease. Release technique got its name because dancers were thought to be "releasing" unnecessary tension by refraining from instructing the body so as to allow forces like gravity to act through them by giving in to momentum. Yet the phrases still signified an artist's unique signature rather than universal kinetic patterns. Nevertheless, the use of anatomical, physical, and mechanical metaphors as teaching tools erased the aesthetic investments of release technique, and the vocabulary was configured as more authentic to the body than the so-called artificiality of modern dance and ballet.

Company dancers teaching set phrases felt they were empowering students based on their own experience of embodying Somatics-informed choreography. For example, Brown's late 1970s and 1980s dancers felt ownership over the vocabulary because they contributed understanding to its execution. Brown did not explain how to execute her work,[129] so in an approach taken up by dancers in other companies,[130] her company turned to Alexander and Klein Techniques for metaphors. Karczag spearheaded the use of Alexander's

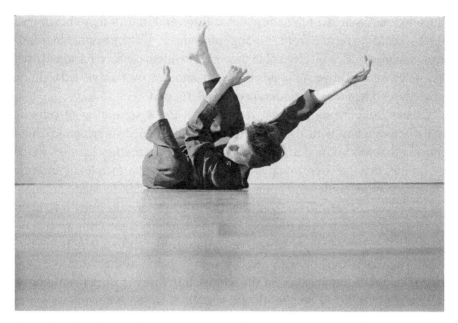

Figure 1.9. Eva Karczag, in the early 1990s, at the European Dance Development Center, Arnhem, Netherlands, where she was a faculty member between 1990 and 2002. Photograph by Nienke Terpsma.

approach after joining the company in the late 1970s.[131] Using what is known as "inhibition," which exhibits similarities to Paxton's ideas about the skills he learned in Tai Chi, Karczag danced using dramatically less effort than she had experienced needing in ballet.[132] She cultivated what she felt was internal space to move with more lyricism, paralleling the reason that 1950s dancers turned to Nikolais's and Hawkins' classes.[133] As a dancer whom Jowitt described as having "graced" Brown's company, Karczag established herself as a master of the choreography through her approach, affirming her creative agency in Brown's work.[134]

Without company class, many of Karczag's colleagues followed her lead.[135] To meet the aesthetic demands of Brown's choreography, they lessened the amount of energy they used, with the aim of curtailing the output of effort that exceeded what they saw as necessary.[136] The idea of overworking, however, carried a more profound significance because it was thought to be a retrogressive psychophysical habit tied up with willful bodily control. Dancers associated the habit with incessant repetition undertaken in modern and classical training, which they viewed as evidence of the authoritarian institution of aesthetics. Dancers therefore invested a sense of empowerment in their approach to the choreography based on Alexander's idea of bringing unconscious capacity under conscious control, and in turn they encouraged their students to refrain from "forcing" movement.[137] Once again, the primitive (unconscious), conceived of in the early twentieth century, reframed itself as a new source of power in opposition with outdated, overly civilized training procedures based on conscious repetitive instruction.

Classes teaching set material recycled the 1960s separation of training and choreography with the belief that students gained information about moving that was not tied to the aesthetics of the phrases they learned. Based on the idea that they were practicing neutral movement principles in set work, students seemed to develop autonomy in these new classes. Madden taught ideas such as counter thrust from Klein's work, in which the body is thought to move away from a direction in which the dancer is connecting with gravitational force.[138] Madden, whom Petronio introduced to Klein Technique when she was struggling with the demands of being in the company, catalyzed the broader application of the approach to Brown's work beginning in the early 1980s.[139] For counter thrust, she aimed to sense moving weight in bony connections, which she also felt augmented the reverberation of movement through the joints as opposed to the classical extension of the limbs. Madden felt that she empowered students by teaching such skills as opposed to having them perform drills of set movement.[140] Kinesthetic awareness, dancers believed, enabled them to make choices based on their unique physical structure rather than simply emulating form. They abandoned the collective exploration of new vocabulary to achieve what they saw as new authority over their craft, reflecting the broader cultural shift toward championing individual initiative.[141]

As approaches based on principles of posture and motion devoid of creative exploration, Alexander's and Klein's techniques lent themselves to the move toward individual autonomy. Fueled by the association with Brown and eventually Petronio, a small New York network developed around the regimens. Klein designed her approach for dancers, but Alexander teachers who were also dancers, such as Remy Charlip, June Ekman, and Marjorie Barstow, all modified the technique for dance. Ekman, who was a revered figure because she had taught Brown, took over a regular class that Charlip had begun, and served several generations of Brown's company as well as other dancers.[142] Karczag introduced new company members to Ekman, who became devotees of the class and also took private lessons.[143] This small community made it possible to bring Barstow to New York for special workshops, who, along with Ekman, was thought to work with greater flow than teachers faithful to Alexander teacher training doctrine.[144]

Through the concept of an integrated body-mind, initially put forward by Alexander but also found in Klein's rhetoric, dancers affirmed the personal significance that set vocabulary had for them. Klein theorized a connection between physical, emotional, and social dimensions, and in Ekman's classes, students felt they were processing emotions, which engendered a private sense of the body that was intertwined with their execution of vocabulary distinct from the choreographer's aims. Despite the embargo on representing emotion, the modern dance idea of expression reframed itself in what was seen as non-expressive material, because dancers felt their skills embodied personal psychophysical truths. As a result, the application of Alexander and Klein Technique to set material further emphasized individuality over collectivity. Even those for whom psychological dimensions were unwelcome followed the trend toward individuality to the degree that they focused on the mastery of complex vocabulary. Receptivity to nature asserted itself anew as the individually potent awareness that could be directed into execution, a value that was reflected in both Alexander's and Klein's class modalities that involved little verbal exchange.

Alongside these changes, the New York East Village community reconfigured rather than disbanded with collectivity. By intentionally distinguishing their approaches from prevailing developments in the field, this small and not necessarily representative group of artists exemplifies the flexibility with which Somatics was instituted. They embraced what had been repudiated in modest performance, forging a milieu that reveled in behaviors not previously acceptable in the modern dance studio. Through the embodiment of emotionality and sexuality, dancers collectively emphasized individual expression. Yet while they critiqued the belief that independence from aesthetics resulted from training based on intrinsic bodily principles, rather than disengaging from the conceit of nature, they reconstructed it by incorporating psychological dimensions. Regimens became popular that combined anatomical images with Jungian symbolism, Eastern mysticism, or other cosmology in procedures that were distinct from both those established in the 1970s and set movement classes. Also, concerned about the imitation that successful Somatics-informed choreography might generate, the dancers marked their creativity with individuality by emphasizing the psychological uniqueness of their exploration.

Thus, beginning in the late 1970s, alongside Brown's first successes on large New York concert stages, East Village dancers sought creative rather than physical autonomy in training directed toward innovation. They embodied radical individuality to critique the conservative cultural agenda intertwined with Reaganomics. Dancers continued to break modern and classical protocols even as they rejected the 1970s conceit of nonaesthetics.

For example, Open Movement, which was neither a dance class nor a performance, fostered exploration similar to early 1960s experimentation.[145] Artists including John Bernd, Stephanie Skura, Mark Russell, Yvonne Meier, Ishmael Houston-Jones, Diane Torr, Tim Miller, and Jennifer Monson gathered at the event that was started by Peter Rose under the influence of Polish theater innovator Jerzy Grotoswki.[146] Artists attending Open Movement contributed to the profile of the East Village as an edgy or risky neighborhood.[147] They integrated language, emotional gesture, and performance art with dance improvisation often involving physical risk.[148] Choreographed references to social and cultural identity exhibited the milieu's vision alongside articles in print media that the community produced, as well as themed concerts and panel discussions.

Many of the dancers felt that Skinner Releasing and Authentic Movement dovetailed with their aims by combining training and creativity. In these regimens, the new significance that sensation had acquired enabled them to reconstruct the body's natural status as unpredictable and emotional. The dancers generated what they felt was idiosyncratic risky dancing based on Skinner's idea that each student must stay true to their indeterminate connection with cosmic forces. Based on the experience of Skinner Releasing, they developed an interest in the individual psychological dancing self, which contributed to the increased popularity of Authentic Movement later in the decade.

Meier initially introduced Skinner's work to her colleagues, who built on and critiqued 1970s ideas using the regimen.[149] Classes often began with the body supine and eyes closed focusing on the kinesthetic awareness of weight, so the format was familiar because all the dancers had taken CI and Anatomical Releasing. Yet, to release tension, for example, Skinner replaced scientific imagery with poetic prompts such as "your bones are melting," which suggested uncertain outcomes from connecting with anatomical function. Kinetic forms and decision-making processes learned in CI informed the dancing, but now in solo, dancers were propelled by the images rather than the moving weight in exchange with a partner. In this sense, the poetic imagery offered a logic different from that of CI to understand the involuntary nature of embodying an established vocabulary. Focused on themselves, students verified the unpredictability of the modality in which they were engaged by moving differently from each other, while with more erratic dancing than that seen in other Somatics classes, they displaced the performance of modesty.[150]

Meier and her colleagues also embraced Whitehouse's theory that the body is the psyche in which social convention prevents authentic motile expression.[151] They felt they were resisting 1980s conservative morality by learning to move without judgment. The integrated body-mind reinvented itself, bringing emotion to the foreground as physical sensation, now understood as unconscious psychological impulses. Dancers moved with eyes closed to enhance their kinesthetic awareness, and primitive psychic impulses sometimes propelled the dancing. In exchanges between a "witness" and mover, participants brought focus to the idea of the psyche,[152] in mediated conversations designed to support the exploration of behavior that would otherwise have seemed inappropriately sexual, aggressive, depressed, afraid, or bored.[153] In activity that resembled popular representations of insane asylums, the dancers resisted concern about their appearance, transgressing the 1980s idealized attractive, high-functioning body. They pressed into each other and the surroundings, repeated actions obsessively, made strange sounds, and threw themselves around.[154] The regular contravention of expressive and relational protocols offered rare social latitude. For example, Jennifer Miller, a woman with a full beard, recalls feeling that her difference did not matter even while her colleagues had an awareness of its significance beyond the rarified East Village milieu.[155] As the culture wars were stirring, the artists asserted their opposition to conservatism with daring, unpredictable dancing, even while they retained a sense of independence from the ideological battles between right and left by remaining true to what they saw as natural psychophysical truths.

In its embrace of Skinner Releasing and Authentic Movement, East Village artists reimagined antiauthoritarianism and the rejection of established aesthetics to respond to changes in the field.[156] They saw Brown's success and elegant seamlessness based on release technique as threatening to the aesthetic protocols they envisioned Somatics as propounding. Furthermore, because their focus resisted conventional virtuosity, the regimens seemed accessible to dancers regardless of prior experience. Rather than pursue the mastery of set material, dancers cultivated psychophysical ease whereby energy purportedly erupted through the body as they submitted to cosmological forces and the unpredictability of the psyche. Class modalities constructed a community of individuals embracing behavior that was not acceptable in 1970s Somatics or 1980s Alexander, Klein, and set movement classes.

The East Village approaches thus benefited from a mystical reconstruction of the natural body, making use of the latest developments in the work of 1970s teachers, in ways that contrasted with the scientific logic of the training applied to set choreography. For example, after initially experimenting with anatomical images, Skinner developed a poetic lexicon that facilitated connection to a cosmological unity.[157] Her images drew on plants, animals, and landscapes, proposing, for example, that bone joints were sea sponges, or legs were shadows falling from a bottomless well at the solar plexus. Through the embodiment of the images, students purportedly reconnected with the collective unconscious, of which the prompts constitute a linguistic form, by translating a felt sense of the body into words. Teachers cultivated receptivity with a hypnotic voice and music, which was thought necessary to embody the ideas that, according to Skinner, must move the dancer rather than being consciously illustrated.[158]

In a related manner, Bainbridge Cohen extended Todd's concept of "form follows function" beyond a conventional scientific construction of the body, even though her lexicon remained anatomical.[159] BMC constructed a body in which the analysis of structure and function focused around the organs, neuroendocrine system, glandular system, fluids, skin, and other "systems," all of which were presumed to contribute to postural and motional hygiene. Because she argued that organs are "primary habitats for emotions, aspirations, and memories," which connect practitioners to "universal symbols and myths," Bainbridge Cohen's concept of nature exhibited the unpredictability that East Village dancers could expand to incorporate affective dimensions.[160] In the throes of BMC procedures, students might burst into tears or enter a panic state, but they were also expected to discover new movement. Bainbridge Cohen conceived of the dancer as entering "the mind" of tissues to access the body's optimum functional and creative potential by listening to corporeality that can, however, never be fully apprehended. The pedagogy therefore urged that teachers attend to students' verbal and nonverbal feedback, following "the mind of the room" with an intuitive attitude about what the body might offer.

To push beyond the scientific rhetoric of the previous decade, 1980s Somatics revisited its representation of East and West, even if these terms were not always used in the teaching language, by using the idea of "energy," which they represented as Eastern. Metaphors such as the chakras were borrowed from South Asian metaphysics, and chi from East Asian medicine. Through these references they intimated a form of knowledge through which to understand bodily experience exceeding Western theories of physics and biology.[161] Based on the synthesis of Somatics and martial arts, dancers also developed teaching practices that emphasized bodily dimensions that Western epistemology purportedly failed to apprehend. For example, Karczag used the Chinese terms yin/yang as an analogy for integrating physical properties that are configured in opposition, proposing that lightness inheres weight and vice versa because gravity entails the counterforce of upward thrust. She also taught Tai Chi as a means to find stillness in movement and vice versa, thereby creating a new mystical version of Paxton's fusion of physics and awareness.[162]

The diversification observable in 1980s Somatics marked a new confidence as the field consolidated. Since the 1970s, Somatics had gained enough traction to sustain greater differentiation broadly defined by, on the one hand, the pursuit of technical mastery of new choreography like Brown's use of Alexander and Klein Techniques and, on the other hand, the cultivation of an unwieldy body that fused Skinner Releasing, Authentic Movement, and BMC with artists' own approaches. At a time when the effects of previous experimentation began infiltrating large concert stages, some dancers reasserted the anti-institutional agency they associated with the natural body. However, many dancers continued to integrate various approaches in their teaching, dancing, and choreography, and the regimens remained largely marginal to and critical of modern and classical approaches. Communities in New York and other large cities supported the development of the field with little institutional support. Yet many dancers disputed the 1970s concept of inclusivity in modes of production, representation, and organization, as the whiteness of Somatics-informed choreography became more and more evident and explicit cultural difference entered the discourse, questioning the proposition that by stripping the body of cultural imposition, one could reveal its natural truth. However, even while Somatics began transforming in line with changing social and artistic circumstances, the idea of a natural body at the center of the training went largely unchallenged as dancers found novel vocabulary in what they believed were previously untapped intrinsic bodily capacities.

Corporate Somatics: Recalibrating Critique for Commercialism

Somatics training in the 1990s felt the increasing corporatization of the arts, both in changes in funding and in a corresponding cultural shift.[163] Exploration dramatically diminished as dance establishments fully endorsed large companies that were influenced by Somatics. To attract sponsorship, programmers promoted artists that had achieved substantial success, so Brown's and Petronio's vocabularies, for example, reached brand-name status within the field. At the same time, arts funding in general diminished, and with fewer funds for experimentation, and therefore woefully little studio time, unknown artists used Somatics ideas to justify relying on dancers to take responsibility for their own training and health, while also asking them to participate more actively in the creative process. Dancers therefore saw their roles reconceived in line with new business management paradigms in which autonomy and responsibility were allegedly enjoyed at all levels of the workforce. Practices, developed as liberatory direct democracy and entrepreneurship only decades before, became new imperatives for employment for both dancers and other workers. Furthermore, even while the art market sought unique choreographic signatures, corporate funding marshaled the homogenization of companies into ones led by an individual, which restored the hierarchy of the choreographer over the dancer, despite the new ways that dancers were being asked to collaborate in the artistic process.

Somatics training, which came increasingly under the jurisdiction of large educational institutions, reflected the reconception of the dancer's role within a corporate logic. Most university dance programs and conservatories embraced Somatics regimens now that they had established themselves on major contemporary dance concert stages. This shift provided employment for artists who were rendered precarious by the paucity of funding for small-scale projects. But education increasingly adopted a business model to compete for enrollment, so teachers were under pressure to market Somatics as valuable for rather than critical of the established field. They reframed the 1970s displacement of authoritarianism and the 1980s critique of universality as valuable pedagogical resources. Yet within the institution, creative and physical autonomy restructured themselves into educational imperatives imposed upon students. Affected by the competitive culture within which Somatics reframed itself, the independent studios of late twentieth-century pioneers also capitalized on the success of companies associated with their approach, promoting their techniques in competition with each other, and with modern and classical trainings.

As part of the revision of Somatics, diversity and ingenuity also reconstructed themselves through new corporate ethics. With artists now pressured to promote a signature, they found that they had to achieve visibility for their creative uniqueness, which some did through initiatives that criticized the performance of modesty. This shift paralleled changes in large businesses, which exploited the creative potential of unique skills found in its workforce, including those that came with differences in genders, races, sexualities, and other social identities.[164] Within the restructuring of organizations, difference and creativity, which had been problematic in the standardizing logic of production lines, became a new imperative for a market thirsty for new products with which to beguile consumers. Dance training institutions followed suit by valuing Somatics regimens thought to teach creative autonomy, while students sought programs that offered choice rather than instituting regimentation. The implementation of Somatics therefore bolstered the idea that academic capitalism offered diversity, choice, and excellence. Similarly, with the growth of the field, professional dancers seemingly had a breadth of choice from which to design training suited to their individual needs and desires. Yet the new corporate logic mediated what they saw as freedom and autonomy, because employment depended on offering flexibility, creativity, and self-responsibility to choreographers running pickup companies with no employment security.[165]

In Somatics training, corporate arts culture overshadowed the collectivism of previous decades, because the regimens became largely associated with aesthetic approaches that were institutionalized by a single artist as either tried and tested or critical and innovative. Somatics no longer signified experimentation now that dancers pursued preexisting images and efficient execution of the moving body through the training. The initial impetus of rejecting training tied to an aesthetic tradition therefore disappeared. Release technique affirmed the homogenization of a dominant look by symbolizing virtuosity associated with Somatics. Such changes erased, for example, how company members, by applying Somatics to the vocabulary, contributed to the conceptualization of Brown's lexicon beginning in the 1970s, because the choreography had now become established as a new style tied to the choreographer. The logic of using set movement in classes therefore shifted from one of practicing skills that offered autonomy to embodying a particular look.[166]

The new corporate arts culture also reframed skills cultivated in Klein and Alexander Techniques. Despite these classes being devoid of dance vocabulary, they were known through their association with large companies, and were therefore seen as serving existing aesthetics. Some of Brown's dancers, for example, felt that Klein training was integral to the vocabulary they performed, so Somatics reconstructed itself as a complement to established aesthetics.[167] Even Skinner Releasing and Authentic Movement linked themselves with artists that achieved visibility through idiosyncratic approaches they had cultivated in the East Village. The East Village milieu, previously critical of the institutionalization of Somatics, now established itself as a launchpad for uptown success. A new generation therefore perceived the regimens as fulfilling the demands of working in an established field rather than a way to explore new choreographic ideas.

The field saw changes in the organizations and the artists offering training, which refigured Somatics as a handmaiden of authorized concert dance rather than a source of innovation. Brown inaugurated ongoing public training at her studio in the 1990s.[168] Somatics formed a significant curricular component, compounding its association with large companies. To teach their regular classes, independent artist-run organizations also increasingly employed dancers working for successful midscale and large companies, including current and ex-dancers for Cunningham, Brown, Bill T. Jones, and Bebe

Miller.[169] Equally important, the companies associated with Somatics began to resemble modern and ballet companies at an organizational level, which affected the training procedures. For example, Brown established her repertory by severing the vocabulary from the dancers on which it was initially made. Successive generations of her company taught the choreography and technique classes and, like their students, brought with them an impetus for pursuing Somatics different from those that had drawn dancers in the previous decades. The idea that accessing individual bodily truths is integral to the pedagogy became generic in the branding of Brown's studio and of Somatics more generally. However, extended periods of sensory focus diminished in classes that now focused on the mastery of set material. Teachers used anatomical terms to explain the movement, much like Schick had pioneered in the 1980s, but without the time to have an individual experience of how a joint moves. Thus, the body constructed itself through the anatomical language as equivalent rather than unique. A tacit rationale became "Everyone can do this movement this way because we all share a common anatomy." Somatics pedagogies therefore transformed themselves yet again to cultivate a look of dancing for the established field, rather than serving as a vehicle promoting individual dance practices.

Even where dancers did sustain a sense of individuality, within a corporate arts culture, such autonomy redefined itself as a means to cultivate excellence as determined by the establishment. Despite the disappearance of reflective time from set classes, some dancers pursued training, like Klein's and Alexander's, which they believed gave them access to a physicality independent of aesthetics by focusing on movement principles.[170] Yet 1990s Somatics approaches reconfigured this separation of training and choreography as a means for dancers to attune their unique bodies to the demands of well-established vocabulary, rather than the logic a decade earlier when dancers had sought strategies to embody new vocabulary.[171] Now dancers looked to autonomy not to divest their dancing of outdated habits and embody novel styles, but to excel in the execution of existing work. For Brown's company, this even extended to dancers aligning their own movement signatures with the idiosyncratic nature of roles that were a legacy of the 1970s and 1980s dancers.[172] At the same time, practitioners still felt that by pursuing training preferences, they were in charge of their bodies, which, by the twenty-first century, extended to classical ballet training for many of Brown's company members.[173]

The emphasis on excellence in fulfilling established vocabulary dovetailed with a re-engagement with classicism. Choreographers like Brown and Petronio integrated classical ideals and employed ballet-trained dancers,

while pedagogy now concerned itself with producing the best, most efficient, and self-sustaining dancers who needed to master extension, elevation,
and balance with precision and clarity of line. Dancers therefore reinhabited
ballet's lexicon rather than extrapolating principles from it as they had in
previous decades. Through the application of Feldenkrais and Alexander
Technique, ballet reconstructed itself as a practice in which autonomy
could be sustained. For example, Luc Venier and Rebecca Nettl-Fiol applied
Alexander Technique to classical training after discovering that "ballet . . . [is]
not divorced from the natural form and function of the self."[174] In the newly
reconstructed ballet, students focused on sensations they attributed to the relationship of physical forces to anatomical structure, so Somatics, which had
historically been thought alien to the external focus demanded by aesthetic
ideals, was no longer seen as oppositional to the classical vocabulary. Ballet
therefore reasserted itself as a ubiquitous foundation and self-evident necessity for training, and aesthetic hierarchies were no longer seen as antithetical
to a dancer's sense of agency.

Now that they were associated with large companies and educational
institutions, the distinct regimens were frequently placed in competition
with each other, which dramatically altered the field. Rather than working as
allies in the development of ideas as they had in the 1970s, many proponents
marketed their approaches to a limited number of influential choreographers,
potential students, and training institutions. A protectionist culture emerged
because the differences between techniques became an important selling
point. In the early 1990s, Skinner and Klein established teacher certification
programs, insisting that their ideas were being watered down by their generic
use.[175] Bainbridge Cohen had been certifying teachers since her first generation of committed students in the early 1970s, but she further consolidated
her technique in the 1990s by publishing *Sensing Feeling and Action*.[176] With
her partner, Barbara Mahler, Klein also copyrighted her technique. The spirit
of investigating gave way to the increasing crystallization of pedagogy, as
proponents disagreed about how to access corporeal authenticity.

Bainbridge Cohen's text powerfully illustrates how practitioners tried to
retain their original intent despite the changes that had occurred since the
1970s. *Sensing Feeling and Action* recasts BMC's collaborative pedagogy as
marketable, yet still affirms the self-reflexive critique of aesthetic ideals at
the heart of the practice. The workbook of exercises maps the body based on
practitioners' common observations, all the while insisting that readers must
trust their own experiences, because new discoveries about unstable, un-
knowable bodily nature are always possible.[177] Bainbridge Cohen therefore
canonizes BMC exploratory pedagogy even while she defers to the absolute

authority of bodily knowledge itself. Similarly, in a collection of essays about Authentic Movement, Whitehouse refers to the limitations of her understanding, which she credits to the growth of the practice and the motion of the psyche.[178] Despite renouncing their jurisdiction, however, both women fixed their ideas with greater sophistication by publishing, which, along with certification programs, intensified the competition between the approaches and resulted in splintering within a regimen as students disagreed with their pioneer-teachers.[179]

Klein and Karczag engaged in a particularly visible struggle because of the association with Brown's company. Klein, promoting her technique, and Karczag, teaching Alexander Technique and Tai Chi, disagreed publicly about how anatomy functions, and therefore how to achieve motile efficiency.[180] Ideological differences fueled the disagreement because Klein seemed to use voluntary control by actively placing and stretching the body. The idea that Brown's dancers were split between the two methods achieved mythic status in the larger Somatics community.[181] Such distinctions proliferated when company dancers pursued teacher training programs because they used the ideas and the terminology they were learning, which contributed to the association of a choreographic style with a particular approach. For example, Brown's dancers Hultman and Senter became certified as Alexander teachers, while Carolyn Lucas and Madden began Klein's teacher training along with Nelson, ex-Cunningham dancer Neil Greenberg, and Ralph Lemon's company dancer Wally Cardona.

Competition between the proponents of the various regimens also dovetailed with and fed upon the institutional embrace of Somatics. Some regimens nevertheless achieved widespread institutionalization as universities and conservatories implemented the approaches to strengthen their training and education. Teachers fought to establish the value of Somatics, arguing for the unique contribution it makes to training dancers and choreographers. For example, permanent and visiting faculty insisted that, as well as cultivating a healthy dancer, Somatics trains the student's body and mind by integrating creativity and training and imparting anatomical information. With the aim of producing the most interesting choreographers and versatile performers, higher education employed dancers who had established a reputation in large companies that were informed by Somatics[182] or were known for iconoclastic choreography.[183] With its teacher certification credential, Skinner Releasing also provided a kind of legitimacy for the academy or conservatory not available through other approaches. Educational institutions affirmed that they offered choice and training excellence with the diverse teaching methods developed in the Somatics field.

As increasingly definitive Somatics pedagogies were marketed in contemporary dance, some veterans in the field feared that the practices in which they had invested so much labor and belief were losing their critical edge. To the degree that release technique signified a recognizable form, it recapitulated modern dance's imposition of aesthetic values. A discourse emerged

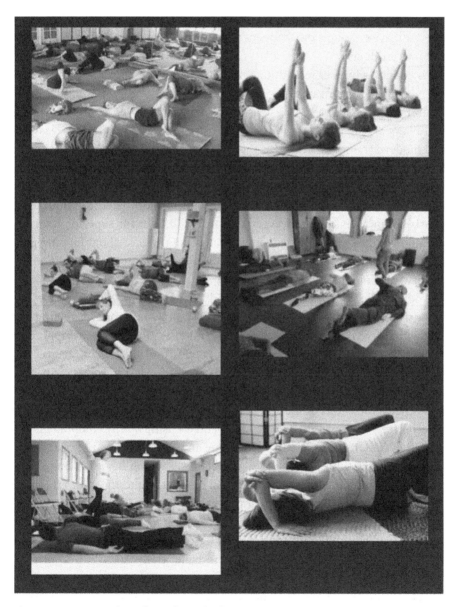

Figure 1.10. Screenshot of search results for "Somatics classes" 2020.

in which imitation of an external form was contrasted with the rigorous and authentic embodiment of Somatics. The quote about faking release, which opened this chapter, exemplifies how dancers opposed imitation to reaffirm the natural basis of Somatics and aspired to ratify its independence from commercial and institutional concerns. Some late twentieth-century pioneers also reassured dancers by accentuating distinctions between their approaches and release technique. The field therefore responded to the impact of corporate culture by reiterating that Somatics allows dancers to access natural creative freedom, even though this happened through the competitive marketing of training products.

As Somatics further institutionalized, it replaced the critique of the establishment with a claim of superiority to compete with modern and classical training. Dancers idealized ease as an experience afforded by the regimens, and blamed injury on the unnecessary use of force. Condemning classical and modern training methods as those that enabled dancers to "fake release," Somatics stood firm on the principle that dancers must cultivate aptitudes to underpin the execution of movement rather than simply copy a form.[184] Each technique asserted its rigor differently, and each negotiated a unique emphasis on an individual process of discovery. To fight for superior status as a training approach, Somatics reinvigorated the rhetoric about tapping into intrinsic bodily capacity now that the value of exploration had diminished in the field of contemporary dance.

Additionally, Somatics rhetoric laid claim to its preeminence by reconstructing bodily nature as a source of moral superiority, equating artistic integrity with the practice of the regimens. Dancers found support in Alexander's, Todd's, and Klein's theories that postural efficiency enhances intellectual, emotional, and spiritual evolution. Furthermore, Todd, Klein, and Bainbridge Cohen naturalized a relationship between anatomical capacity and other dimensions of the self by arguing that efficiency and coordination reverberate on all levels of being and depend on using bodily components for what they are intended.[185] Klein technique and BMC equated physical depth of bodily tissues with psychological corollaries.[186] Klein held that bony connection engenders a "knowing state," which is the highest goal of art, while Bainbridge Cohen's "state of knowing" depended on the "centering" of awareness with action. Dancers believed that working with superficial muscle resulted in injury and indicated a lack of personal and artistic integrity;[187] the modalities in "fake" release, modern, and ballet trainings thus purportedly resulted in arrested development.

At the same time, and in spite of the social stratification that Somatics pedagogies had sustained, black and other nonwhite artists, and dancers with sexual identities that seemed to contravene the aim of bodily purity, appropriated the regimens away from their exclusionary roots.[188] Many artists refused to take the rhetoric of different regimens as credo, extracting the value they found while discarding other information. Meier exhibited this strategy, for example, by continuing to use Skinner Releasing despite identifying its limits. Movement Research, the independent training organization started in the East Village, also helped to position Somatics as training that served the political aims of diversity by programming teachers working with the regimens alongside non-Western training.[189] All these changes provided some reassurance for the field, which had become noticeable for its exclusivity in the 1980s, not least through the choreographic interventions of African American and queer artists.

By identifying what they took from Somatics, dancers reassured themselves that they were not faking release, and that they had an edge over those following more traditional training. For example, at a time when artistic and physical integrity seemed to be in short supply because of the potential to fake release, dancers fed their nostalgia for a time before corporate Somatics by taking classes with veterans in the field, who signified the uncompromising experimentation of earlier decades. With an exploratory pedagogy connected to their improvisational practices, artists such as Paxton, Karczag, Simone Forti, Lepkoff, Nelson, and Nancy Stark Smith supplied a noticeable alternative to Somatics efficiency and proficiency. Their artistic histories and reputations as performers bolstered the sense that their classes granted a unique take on the body, affirming the potency of Somatics. And again, when dancers taught the 1970s and 1980s repertory, which was originally choreographed on them, they endowed students with the feeling of accessing the source of vocabulary that had now achieved brand status. Karczag, Kraus, Shick, and Madden, as well as Forti, taught in institutional and other settings, bringing their original vision of the choreography, and therefore rejuvenating its artistic value.[190] Finally, certain practitioners gained notoriety for being able to arouse the body's intrinsic capacities in one-to-one hands-on sessions. Dancers praised the "good hands" of Klein, Karczag, Bainbridge Cohen, Ekman, and the BMC teacher Beth Goren. Pursuing individual sessions with these teachers, dancers contrasted the depth and integrity of their work to the superficiality of copying the forms called release technique.

Benefiting from the diversity of approaches in the field at the end of the twentieth century, dancers sought both the creative skills necessary to contribute to choreography and the dexterity, sustainability, and self-responsibility necessary for employment in a company. Yet the regimens no longer represented a break from modern dance, or even the critique of 1970s aesthetics, but instead guaranteed the skills necessary for the job market. To the degree that Somatics achieved significance either for its role in dancers' health and sustainability or for engendering creativity, the belief that the regimens furnished contemporary dance with a new comprehensive training all but died. Most dancers and educators came to see Somatics as a complement to other training. Despite such dramatic change, and even though the regimens had become increasingly distinct and competitive, a natural body still asserted itself as central to the training. Dancers believed they were accessing the same functional imperatives in distinct ways in the various regimens, for different purposes. For example, they saw themselves as accessing essential bodily truths by engaging kinesthetic awareness differently in distinct techniques. Thus, the tropes, language, and conception of sensation all pointed to common intrinsic bodily principles.

Conclusion

With the enduring belief that Somatics enabled them access to the body's authentic and inherent nature, dancers affirmed that the corporeal material at the center of their art form was precultural and transhistorical. Yet the development of the regimens over the last four decades of the twentieth century reveals the cultural labor through which this idea of nature was constructed. The procedures and vocabularies through which dancers found a bodily truth exhibited substantial change, along with the organization of classes and the rhetoric through which Somatics was framed. The 1970s saw students cultivating kinesthetic awareness, explored in pedestrian-like vocabulary. Practitioners believed they were sensing the action of physical forces through the skeleton in neutral and innate movement that connected them to human evolutionary heritage. The simplicity of practice, compared with other training, engendered antihierarchical collectivism in a culture of willing exchange, both within and beyond the studio. By the next decade, however, many dancers had disbanded with ordinary movement and collective ethics to pursue individual goals in classes that still proffered kinesthetic awareness of functional imperatives as a foundation but entailed reproducing novel complex set choreography. Meanwhile, artists that sustained the 1970s impulse of resisting institutionalized aesthetics did so by arguing that emotional and sexual impulses, overlooked by their predecessors, were integral to bodily nature, and this resulted in a greater emphasis on individuality in vigorous and jarring vocabulary that appeared idiosyncratic compared with pedestrian movement. Toward the end of the twentieth century, the agency that dancers had enjoyed through asserting staunch individualism collapsed. Now marshaled by corporate arts culture, the natural body reconstructed itself as a source of artistic and moral superiority, serving dancers who executed vocabulary into which classical and modern lexicons had been integrated. The regimens competed for preeminence as a training approach by defining themselves against techniques that were seen as compromising the dancer's artistic integrity.

Despite such dramatic changes, dancers sustained their belief in the natural status of the body by directing their attention away from the social and economic conditions affecting their practice and toward a timeless corporeality defined by primitive, scientific, and mystical properties. With romanticized and idealized visions of other cultures, species, and stages in human development, cultures that were represented as Eastern or primitive, along with children and animals, served as an undifferentiated counterpoint to Western ideologies and morals. Somatics discourse also erased its historical and cultural specificity through recourse to scientific rhetoric, which was presented as factual proof of the mystical insights drawn from Eastern traditions and the basic principles found in atavistic corporeality. The body therefore was constructed to serve as an invisible category of nature that nevertheless perpetrated privilege and exclusion, even while it claimed to be universal.[191]

Yet even though the concept of the natural body depended on exclusionary rhetoric, dancers undeniably achieved various kinds of progressive agency through the training. In Somatics they found evidence that the available knowledge about dance failed to apprehend the complexity of the body that teachers used to modulate training and take greater care of their students. As explored in chapter 3, artists used the sense of self they constructed in Somatics to project their identities beyond the limits of existing gender, race, sexuality, and disability discourses in a manner similar to midcentury artists. However, to the degree that Somatics postulated the possibility of transcending sociohistorical limitations by connecting with the body's essence, it naturalized an American postwar liberal ideal of universal individual freedom. As this liberal ideology ascended and transformed throughout the late twentieth century, it helped to conceal the impact of changing economic and cultural conditions upon the regimens, because along with contemporary dance, Western societies sought universal individual freedom on a much broader level. The limits and possibilities of the idea of nature came into view when Somatics reached other national and regional contexts, and American specificity was challenged and transformed, as we will see in the next chapter.

2

Contradictory Dissidence

Somatics and American Expansionism

Although dancers using Somatics were critical of American cultural dominance and mainstream cultures generally, as well as their perceived artistic constraints, they nonetheless embodied American cultural expansionism in a transnational context. Incorporating the post–World War II ideology of the United States as the center of a Western culture in which artists were purportedly free to push against institutionalized aesthetics and dominant values, dancers throughout the 1970s and 1980s forged a transnational community that saw itself as resisting the dominance of American modern dance. Through a loose network of independent artists and organizations, as well as isolated institutions, Somatics reached hubs in Britain, the Netherlands, and Australia, as well as basing itself in New England. New York established itself as the origin of the training, compounding the idea that the United States was the center of a Western culture that protected the universal right to individual freedom against fascist and communist regimes. Although highly significant, German modern dance's influence on the regimens all but disappeared into the impression that the training was imported from America.[1] Isolated artists and teachers working in all the locales outside of the United States prior to the 1960s also contributed to the domestic impact of Somatics and modern dance. Yet the symbolic centrality of New York largely erased these histories. Ideas seemed to flow outward from America's cultural capital, which compounded expansionism.[2]

The charge that 1970s Somatics embodied American expansionism will seem like a stretch to anyone aware of the meager resources to which artists had access, compared with the power behind US foreign policy. Since the 1950s, the government and industries had ploughed capital into military, economic, and cultural expansion, yet educators and artists patchworked together a Somatics network through personal connections based on artistic commitment and goodwill. A handful of dancers initially disseminated Somatics, which illustrates the small scale on which they were working.[3] Americans teaching Somatics in England through a festival at Dartington

The Natural Body in Somatics Dance Training. Doran George, Oxford University Press (2020). © Oxford University Press.
DOI: 10.1093/oso/9780197538739.001.0001.

College of the Arts, for example, were paid little more than travel. However, to garner support, British, along with Dutch and Australian, dancers linked their work with America's position as a center of Western culture, a logic through which a handful of American dancers also secured jobs in Dutch and British higher education. Americans visiting the Dartington festival also taught at local independent collectives where they verified their artistic merit even if they earned little money. In all cases, Somatics found new devotees, while extending America's centrality.[4]

Those who disseminated Somatics beyond New York probably gained some of their confidence based on their knowledge of Cunningham's ascendency. After being denied state funding and access to prestigious venues in New York, Cunningham received highly enthusiastic responses for his independently funded 1964 London engagement. By conquering British conservatism, Cunningham inaugurated his artistic dissidence while questioning the New York establishment's commitment to artistic freedom.[5] Cunningham represented an individual who overstepped domestic cultural limitations, and thereby demonstrated that America lacked communist and fascist repression. His success seemed to prove that America produces dissident choreographers expressing international rather than domestic concerns. For artists who were aware of his struggles with the establishment, and many associated with Somatics were his dancers or mentees, Cunningham symbolized artistic integrity, which he verified internationally through an iconoclastic and therefore dissident venture.[6]

To the degree that Somatics-based artists critiqued the widespread institution of American modern dance, artists seemed to reject American cultural dominance, so American expansionism seemed to be absent from the project of dissemination. Dancers also saw their work as being culturally independent because of the rhetoric claiming that the training accesses neutral bodily imperatives. Yet native avant-gardes that formed outside of the United States often depended on American creative and pedagogical resources to fight structural exclusion from their own dance establishments. As it came into contact with specific conditions, Somatics manifested in different ways through the renewable originality of the universal-individual nature articulated in chapter 1. The plasticity of the Somatics tropes overshadowed American cultural dominance and obscured the impact of local circumstances on the regimens.

In different hubs, the ideal of individual creative freedom dovetailed with local artistic and social development. This chapter therefore begins in the United States, with an analysis of both New York City and New England as distinctive sites of Somatics practice. It then makes a whirlwind tour of Britain, the Netherlands, and Australia, to look at how artists staged critique and adapted Somatics to changing circumstances. We will visit New York artists who opposed the establishment's commitment to 1940s modernism, along-side a New England culture that claimed to provide respite from the demands of professionalism. We then take a trip to London, where dancers infused Somatics with feminist ideals against the local demand for classical virtuosity and what was seen as the American penchant for abstraction. Dutch educators insisted that by instituting Somatics, their training was at the forefront of in-novation, unfettered by the commercialism of any professional dance context, whereas Australian dancers pursued Somatics, in part as a training for decol-onization from European aesthetics.

In my analysis, geography occupies a symbolic as much as factual role be-cause the signifying agency of place is inextricable from the material and his-torical conditions through which the differently located artists and practices contributed to the transnational discourse. I hypothesize five geo-Somatics bodies, bodies resulting from the practice of Somatics in distinctive geo-graphical locales, to represent ideas that emerged as dancers negotiated diverse local conditions while also responding to New York's cultural dom-inance. The scope of this project prevents me from accounting for the com-plexity of each locale. Nevertheless, the regional distinctiveness finds expression in the relationships between institutions and independent artists, and the emergence of artists' organizations and publications. Such signifi-cance either resonated throughout the whole network or between select hubs or was only important locally. The character of all geo-Somatics bodies was evident in every locale. However, New York's dominance meant that it often failed to acknowledge non-American contexts in the way that it represented the variety of ideas. British colonialism and European proximity also compli-cated the exchanges between Britain, the Netherlands, and Australia. Despite contradictions, exceptions, and unevenness, I believe that the geo-Somatics bodies still represent the most accurate version of the discourse that emerged within the transnational community.

Building as it did upon the dissemination of modern dance, the trans-national discourse of Somatics had historical precedents in each locale. New York Somatics symbolized "innovation and professionalism," because the contemporary use of Somatics seemed to originate in this city. British artists emphasized "political and socially signifying" Somatics fueled by am-bivalence toward New York formalism, and by their response to their own conservative dance establishment. Dutch Somatics secured itself as a body "in flux" in dance education, rejecting preexisting vocabulary, which exhibited the aversion to imitation central to midcentury American modern dance.

Cultural independence in the 1970s contributed to "new frontier" Australian Somatics in which natural propensities were in part thought to liberate domestic dance from European traditions.

For each site, I examine the character of the organizations that formed to manage training, concerts, and other activity, along with artists' experiences of the different locales between which they moved. By assessing the impact of local concert dance history and sociopolitical circumstances, I analyze artists' accounts of the countries in which they worked and the means by which organizations fulfilled a particular role. For example, I compare how organizations represented themselves in their publications, what kinds of activities they undertook, and how these factors changed over time, as well as how local publications represented other sites in the network. The geo-Somatics bodies developed their definitions through dancers' ideas about what they were doing and the ethics and protocols of organizations. However, the distinct contextual character of the regimens also reveals how expansionist liberalism manifested through the artistic and sociopolitical histories of a locale, as well as how it was impacted by the relationships between different nation states.

New York Somatics: Innovation and Professionalism

To achieve its centrality to transnational Somatics, New York built on its reputation as epitomizing American high culture. It relied on a discourse constructed by commentators and patrons in major Western centers that depended on establishing national specificity while claiming to address international rather than domestic concerns.[7] With an arts milieu that critiqued mainstream and establishment values, New York held exceptional status in the United States as a center for postwar cultural dissidence. The city's modern dance avant-garde fulfilled postwar high-culture ideals through a critique of the structural imposition of establishment modernism and a questioning of the idea that choreography should speak to the suburban middle classes.[8] Repudiating virtuosity and also the communicative transparency achieved with theatrical themes like Graham's, artists such as Forti, Paxton, Brown, and others intertwined artistic dissidence with elitism.[9] Yet dancers also sought institutional recognition to prove their credibility against any limitations that might be placed on what constituted modern dance. The city therefore became known for both innovation and professionalism.

The impression that Somatics flowed out of New York to other contexts built upon a pattern already established in modern dance. Students had traveled from abroad to New York to train at least since the 1950s, and the United States had also vigorously exported modern dance beginning in 1954 as part of its Cold War diplomacy. The reputation that Judson Church fast achieved as a flashpoint in contemporary dance also underlined New York's symbolic significance. Many of the American practitioners of Somatics who initiated the transnational network participated in or identified with the Judson Church milieu, and the regimens were often taught in conjunction with ideas to which it was linked.[10] The first published writing about major departures from established modern dance also focused on artists associated with Judson. These texts quickly reached Anglophone contexts beyond America as well as the Netherlands.[11] Therefore, even when there was awareness of the range of influences, New York claimed the status of updating and consolidating Somatics. For example, Pauline De Groot, who first introduced the regimens to the Netherlands, imported a variety of influences including Hawkins's and Halprin's approaches. Yet when Contact Improvisation (CI) dancer David Woodberry demonstrated the improvised duet form in her Amsterdam studio, De Groot associated the new vocabulary with Judson experimentation.[12] Similarly, Anatomical Releasing, Forti's work, and that of Lisa Nelson, who started in CI but developed her own sensory-based approach, all acquired an association with Judson's watershed aesthetics when they first reached foreign hubs. New York's significance dominated the understanding of how Somatics developed, sometimes framing artists who were not currently or had never been based in the city, and overshadowing historical and geographic diversity.[13]

New York Somatics positioned its pedagogy as an innovative source of professional excellence when concert dance values began to change in the 1980s. For example, the British press reception of Brown rapidly changed from dismissive to adulatory in the early 1980s, and programmers for London's large "Dance Umbrella" festival began programming artists like Paxton.[14] Yet while this established some legitimacy for Somatics on British stages, the major dance training institutions still primarily implemented Graham, Cunningham, and ballet techniques, as did their American corollaries. In marginal contexts, however, because dancers had access to artists such as Kraus and Paxton who were seen on large stages, they had insider knowledge on the approaches being endorsed by the establishment through the pedagogy and studio performances.[15] After dancing for Brown, Stephen Petronio swiftly followed in her footsteps with his own company, being presented at Dance Umbrella in the 1980s. Like Brown, his dancers taught in marginal contexts, thereby promoting the image of Somatics as both innovative and professional.[16]

As the century progressed, emerging East Village dance contributed to New York's significance by implementing Somatics in ways that seemed oppositional to the aesthetics that were gaining recognition. Along with Ishmael Houston-Jones, Stephanie Skura, Yvonne Meier, and Jennifer Monson, whose training innovations I detailed in chapter 1, Pooh Kaye and others used the regimens to develop explosive, awkward, and bound movement.[17] Critics read the vocabularies as violent compared with the easy, seamless dancing that had become associated with Somatics. A 1986 reviewer refers to "the artfully disheveled dancers [who] slam, bang, smash, heap, tussle and grapple" in Houston-Jones's *Them*.[18] London withheld from these artists the kind of embrace it offered to the other New Yorkers I have mentioned, but Dutch education exploited the critique Houston-Jones, Meier, Monson, Skura, and others offered as guest teachers. Equally important, a small community of marginal British artists identified with the East Village against London's approved version of experimentation.[19] New York therefore sustained its claim to fomenting greater innovation than other contexts.

All in all, New York established itself as an origin for successive waves of dynamic, innovative, and contradictory implementations of the regimens. Practitioners from across the transnational network viewed the city as home to the most advanced experimentation. In her documentation of 1970s and

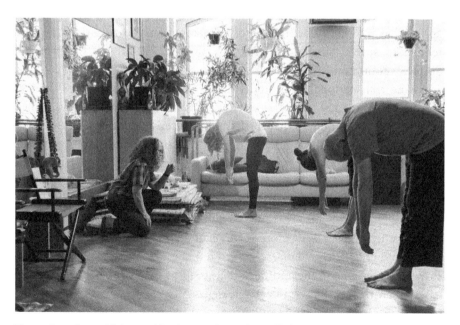

Figure 2.1. Susan Klein teaching her students the "roll-down" in 2015.
Photograph by Brittany Carmichael.

early 1980s British dance, Stephanie Jordan, for example, recalls that "for several years American work [primarily coming from New York] dominated Dance Umbrella if only because it seemed so fresh . . . clearly breaking ground in comparison with most British work." Many of the artists to whom Jordan refers contributed to the development of Somatics.[20] New York thus saw a heavy traffic of dancers from Britain, but also the Netherlands and Australia, all seeking the latest developments. The city became something of a gateway for approaches to the rest of the network, compounding its status as the origin for the regimens even though Somatics drew upon myriad influences from across and beyond the United States such as the West Coast, the Midwest, and Germany. [21]

New York's function as a Somatics mecca meant that approaches launched in the city rapidly achieved transnational dissemination.[22] Resident New Yorkers applied the techniques to choreography that was more likely to reach national and foreign audiences than work from other hubs, exemplified in the ways that Alexander and Klein Techniques became prominent through their association with Brown and Petronio. Furthermore, visiting regional American and foreign dancers brought home the techniques they encountered in New York. Teachers who developed Somatics in other contexts failed to achieve significance to the same degree as New Yorkers unless they established a Manhattan presence.[23] A New York timeline for the application and popularity of techniques therefore had enormous influence on the use of approaches in other hubs. Techniques developed in non-American contexts tended to spread slowly or remained marginal within the transnational Somatics community.[24]

As the transnational community accessed different approaches through New York, Somatics from the city acquired the association with professionalism despite the fact that distinct aims often underpinned New York's dancers' use of the techniques. The non-American hubs encountered the different regimens in close proximity. So along with the common kinetic and textual metaphors, the timeline on which different techniques reached beyond America overshadowed the different artistic strategies in New York Somatics.[25] Paxton and Forti first taught improvisational approaches in Europe only a few years before Kraus had students learning Brown's choreography, and British dancers connected the skills necessary to execute Brown's material with the aptitudes that underpinned CI, which is why they came up with the term "contact release."[26] Most commentators on British dance still associate Paxton, Fulkerson, and the various American teachers at the Dartington festival with a common approach.[27] Despite the divergent projects from which, for example, CI and Brown's concert stage choreography emerged, dancers connected commercial success with investigative processes, which the common association with Judson affirmed. Consequently, innovation and professionalism were fused in the transnational significance of New York Somatics.[28]

Notwithstanding the foreign misrecognition of similarities between contrasting approaches, New York's material circumstances also fomented a connection between innovation and professionalism. New York's dancers enjoyed the opportunity to commit themselves to Somatics to a greater degree than those in other contexts. The high levels of interest granted teachers the opportunity to tailor classes and scheduling to provide regular training for dancers, including the translation of regimens not originally designed for dance. Dancers capitalized on the available resources including training as teachers of Somatics while performing, which, as the field developed, resulted in the knitting together of the regimens with new choreography such as Brown's and Petronio's. All in all, the application of Somatics to dance was seen to have reached levels of sophistication in New York that were not possible in hubs with smaller communities using the regimens.

New York's unmatched volume of activity engendered a rich discourse as artists discussed the value of regimens for distinct professional demands. To the degree that Manhattan saw choreography that was influenced by various regimens, dancers exchanged ideas and disagreed about their experience of the training. Such a focus contrasted with Britain, the Netherlands, and Australia, where pioneers had to fight to establish a place for Somatics within newly emerging modern dance scenes or rationalize the value of the training for higher education. The students populating classes that artists ran independently in the non-American sites sometimes came in search of "New Age" culture and had little interest in professional dance, and often limited experience.[29] The historical unevenness in modern dance therefore meant that beyond New York, Somatics lacked the same focus on professional dance.

Professionalism also asserted itself through New York dancers' choice to continue training in ballet alongside Somatics. Klein Technique, which was strongly associated with New York and secured its professionalism by its 1990s affiliation to Brown and Petronio,[30] was used by those companies' dancers to cultivate precision, endurance, extension, and elevation while sustaining the connection to gravity that is so central to Somatics. So while sharing principles with other approaches, Klein insisted her training applied to all styles, which spoke to New Yorkers who continued to train classically.[31] Her technique ascended in the 1990s as part of the diminishment of a distinction between Somatics-informed vocabulary and classical and modern dance, which I will address in chapter 3. In the 1990s Klein Technique also asserted exceptional professionalism by distinguishing itself from "releasing," and thereby disowning the rejection of modern and classical aesthetics on which most Somatics was initially based.[32]

Even East Village artists, who critiqued the vocabularies on large concert stages and resisted commercialism, still focused on professionalism by stripping Somatics of its association with personal development. Dancers in New England and those in the CI network cultivated therapeutic community with the psychological emphasis in Body-Mind Centering (BMC) and Authentic Movement, and also for CI dancers when improvising in their duet form. For example, 1987 subscribers to *Contact Quarterly (CQ)* read a talk on "Physical Movement and Personality" by Mary Starks Whitehouse, an editorial decision that supports Cynthia Novack's conviction that dancers largely acknowledged the therapeutic benefits of dancing CI.[33] Arguing that this understanding was heightened in the mid-1980s, she quotes a practitioner who "suggested that contact 'puts you in touch with something experienced as a child with a parent--it's a nurturing kind of dance.'"[34] By strong contrast, Houston-Jones, Monson, and Meier, in particular, used the same techniques in the 1980s to create confrontational artistic products, which, while challenging the aesthetics that were becoming institutionalized, did so as a provocative theatrical force.

Also largely an East Village endeavor, Movement Research, from its 1970s beginnings, exhibited a combined emphasis on professionalism and innovation in the use of Somatics.[35] Started as a collective service organization, Movement Research initially consolidated the field simply by registering the classes, workshops, and other information pertaining to artists' independent activity, a function not dissimilar to the one that *CQ* fulfilled.[36] Yet it grew exponentially throughout the 1980s, accessing larger amounts of funding, programming its own daily technique classes and workshops, and organizing performances and public symposia and hiring an executive director.[37] Through its prominence in New York dance as well as shaping the debate with the topics of discussion put forward, Movement Research validated the teachers and dancers it selected, because being programmed by the organization came to signify having achieved a level of success. From a collective of artists sharing information about classes, Movement Research ultimately established a legitimizing role for itself. Yet, unlike many other collectives initiated in the 1970s, the organization remained under artists' creative control, sustaining its reputation as supporting innovation.[38]

From the 1970s onward, artists who linked themselves with New York City gained employment in all the transnational hubs.[39] Relationships forged in New York signified a shared understanding about dance, which contributed to the dissemination of Somatics. Educators secured positions in higher education by word of mouth, through connections made in or associated with New York.[40] Loose networks also increasingly thrived based on time dancers had spent in New York or through personal connections they had with artists from the city.[41] Artists who were isolated in their domestic contexts affirmed the value of their endeavors with the festival community, while New York Somatics functioned as the referent for what put them at odds at and with home. For artists fighting with their domestic establishments, the city symbolized the potential for the fruition of dissident projects.

With its self-image as the center of innovation and professionalism, New York was largely oblivious to the geo-Somatics bodies in transnational contexts beyond America. Yet because dancers depended on proving an international rather than domestic focus of their work, Britain and Holland were important for New Yorkers.[42] Artists that were not circulating in large concert spaces simultaneously verified their resistance toward domestic mainstream values and their international relevance by teaching and performing for small-scale foreign organizations.[43] With paid employment abroad, New Yorkers affirmed their cutting-edge status while earning revenue and the confidence to pursue their work and establish significance at home. Yet they only seemed to notice European dance when it posed competition for the symbolic status of their city as the center of innovation.[44] Foreign artists rarely taught in New York, which may reflect the city's belief in its creative superiority, but could also be because British, Dutch, and Australian levels of state funding were higher than those in America. The resources were likely more available to fly Americans to foreign contexts, and artists abroad were less able to seek teaching opportunities in New York. Nevertheless, and for whatever reasons, the disparity in who was teaching where contributed to the direction of ideas outward from New York.

In the final analysis, New York's innovative and professional Somatics body cannot be separated from accelerated commercialization in the field beginning in the 1970s. The early 1960s anti-virtuoso projects avoided large concert venues, but by the late 1970s artists who had engaged in such experimentation, such as Brown and Childs, both choreographed Somatics into a new virtuosity in major theaters.[45] As I detail in chapter 1, this change in contexts dovetailed with the increasing use of commercial and institutional structures by artists and teachers to expand their projects, contributing to the impressive diversity of techniques that New York housed from the 1980s onward. Creativity therefore linked itself with commercial success in New York Somatics, and thus the natural body presented itself as a site of mutual cocreation between individual freedom and capitalist industry, engendering a key principle of American liberalism. As we will see, with New York's significance as the center of the transnational network, the Somatics bodies in all the other hubs emerged in relation to the naturalization of this expansionist ideology.

New England Somatics: Artistic Respite

New England Somatics positioned itself against its New York equivalent. Beginning in the 1970s, dancers and educators constructed a conception of the body associated with rural living that purportedly recuperated integrity, an essential aspect of innovation. This integrity was seen as having been thwarted and curtailed by commercialism and professionalism. Thus, they rejected the conventional ideas about success to which New York Somatics had become tied, and focused on rigorous experimentation, fending off the encroachment of the dance establishment and mainstream culture. These artists participated in the cultural dissidence associated with the 1970s "back to the land" movement, which Dona Brown describes as the symbolic exodus of white, middle-class Americans to rural environments, renouncing the mainstream culture of commercially dominated environments.[46] She notes, in *Back to the Land*, that aiming to escape the suburbs with which they associated "mindless consumerism and a soul-destroying culture of conformity[,] . . . back-to-the-landers . . . perceived a return to the land as safeguarding their personal and political independence."[47] By rejecting prevailing expectations about how ordinary people organize their lives, dancers and other back-to-the-landers not only asserted their right to go against the grain but also reanimated a key tenet of liberalism in which the individual must be protected from unchecked commerce.[48]

Almost all of the artists living in New England retained a relationship with dance in New York and depended on employment in higher education for income as well as opportunities to develop their ideas. Paxton, Forti, Lepkoff, Nelson, and Deborah Hay all based themselves in rural Vermont and neighboring states, while in Northampton, Massachusetts, Bainbridge Cohen relocated her school for BMC, and Nancy Stark Smith inaugurated *CQ*. Yet many of these artists retained real estate in New York, and they all kept artistic connections with the city.[49] Nevertheless, along with some independent activity, artists found employment at Bennington and the Five Colleges among other university dance programs, and New England Somatics established a semiautonomous network with distinct values. Artists based in the region encouraged their university students to do their own research rather than training them for existing companies, while New York–based dancers escaped north to recuperate from the demands of the city by "rediscovering their natural integrity."

Other regions around the United States held similar symbolic significance, but the proximity of New England to New York afforded it a privileged position in the transnational network. The University of Illinois functioned as an important hub while Skinner was there, and when she subsequently based her training in Seattle, the association of the city with nature contributed to the understanding of her technique.[50] In contrast, San Francisco spawned a Somatics body that, through its interface with the city's "sex positive" culture, diverged dramatically from the implementation of the regimens in both New York and New England.[51] Yet to the degree that the aim of respite from professionalism demonstrates regional variation in American Somatics, New England is undoubtedly the most vivid and influential example.

Somatics and the 1970s back-to-the-land movement shared the construction of nature in a number of ways that seemed to make the connection between artistic integrity and rural living indisputable. For practitioners in both cultures, naturalness signified a timeless but also novel solution to the problems of contemporary life. Similarly to Somatics, which obscured the ways that it drew on ideas from earlier eras, the back-to-the-land movement constructed respite in nature as being newly discovered.[52] They used late nineteenth-century ideas that one can escape from the ills of capitalism through rural self-sufficiency, paralleling their dancing contemporaries who drew on the Progressive Era idea that restoring natural propensities overcomes the ill effects of Victorian deportment.[53] Dancers and back-to-the-landers reconstructed existing ideas of nature to find a sense of personal authenticity that afforded spiritual rejuvenation and constituted political activism.[54] The two movements shared the conviction that reconnecting with an essential way of living restores personal autonomy. Etched, as it was, into the history of modern dance and the American Left, the metaphor of nature appeared self-evident as a means by which to escape contemporary disillusionment. For dancers, rural and provincial New England thereby presented itself as a garden to reconnect with bodily nature, unfettered by the social complexities of New York.

To construct New England Somatics, dancers sustained the trope of iconoclasm that had established itself in postwar modern dance and was also key for the back-to-the-land movement. With so many Americans dreaming of rural living without the means or commitment to do so, some of those who succeeded achieved mythic status as examples to whom others could look.[55] Similarly, artists living in remote New England became iconic as flouting the need for success. Through "opting out," well-known New Englanders sustained a New York presence, signifying integrity for dancers in the city.[56] Artists in remote locations seemed to cultivate practice that was less affected by the problems of professional dance, such as those that arose in the 1980s when dancers first became concerned that Somatics was losing critical potential through imitation of a "release style." The symbolic value of rural living contributed to the reputation of artists like Paxton and Forti who cultivated unique practices in their solo improvising and teaching. As the century progressed, New England Somatics therefore provided a home for 1970s-style investigation that was increasingly displaced by the repetition of set choreography.[57] Images of agrarian lifestyles entered the language of training through the idea that ongoing labor in rural living is dictated by the seasons, which parallels the Somatics idea that bodily authenticity and autonomy are "recovered" through connecting with natural imperatives.[58] Artists also changed the organization of concerts to emphasize the act of dancing over the design of choreography, stressing that the performers were in tune with natural imperatives that could not be contained by tightly defined compositional structures.

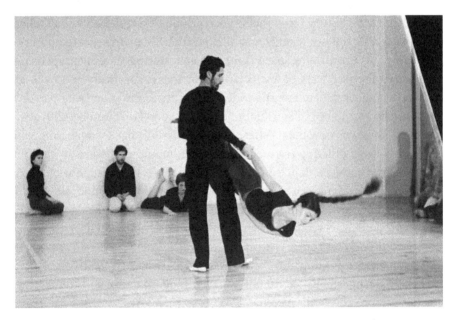

Figure 2.2. Steve Paxton and Nancy Stark Smith in Northampton, Massachusetts, performing with Freelance Dance, a company formed by Lisa Nelson, Danny Lepkoff, and Christina Svane, who are watching. 1980.
Photograph by Stephen Petegorsky.

Much like the fantasy of living beyond the reaches of the state and capitalism, however, the idea of working beyond the clutches of commercialism and the institution was mostly symbolic. To sustain a rural dance practice most often required either independent wealth or a substantial income that did not impose the time constraints of most conventional employment.[59] Consequently, some New York dancers behaved like tourists, leaving the city for short periods with romantic notions of what the land had to offer, rarely confronting its often harsh realities. Capitalizing on the idea of rural respite, they organized and attended Somatics workshops in New England, yet they remained connected with metropolitan art worlds. Paxton, for example, who actually ran a farm, continued to be employed throughout the transnational network after moving to rural Vermont in the 1970s, an experience that contrasts with Skura's, who found that when she moved to the countryside around Seattle in the 1990s, sustaining the level of interest in her work that she had enjoyed in New York became increasingly hard.[60] The disparity in their experiences probably reflects the difference in their status, because unlike Skura's position as a second-generation experimental artist, Paxton rapidly came to be seen as a pioneer and an icon of new practices associated with Judson and then CI. However, regardless of the realities of artists' lives, by signifying the return to the body's essence, New England Somatics established a unique character for itself.

Distinctions between the Massachusetts-based *CQ* and Movement Research exemplify some concrete effects of the divergence between New York and New England Somatics. Both organizations started in the 1970s as registers for classes, but when Movement Research began programming, its relationship to its artistic community contrasted with that of the New England publishers known as Contact Editions. Dancers had started *CQ* to avoid professionalizing CI, whereas Movement Research, as I argued in chapter 1, moved toward professionalization.[61] Novack points out that influential figures in CI exerted influence through *CQ*, which allowed them to avoid copyrighting the form or establishing teacher accreditation, because through the articles they published, dancers were directed toward an idea of good practice, and the register tracked the developing community.[62] The events *CQ* listed also tended to invite participation regardless of dancers' level of experience, which differed from the professional program Movement Research advertised and ultimately offered. Furthermore, while contributors to *CQ* wrote about the therapeutic aspects of CI and Somatics, *Movement Research Performance Journal (MRPJ)* primarily focused on professional training or performance, albeit for many dancers who likely struggled to make a living at their craft. Some of these differences probably arose because the journals, being cognizant of each other and sharing some readership, aimed to sustain a distinction. What is more, the contrast between the two organizations was anything but clear cut because East Villagers participated in the CI network.[63] However, it is fair to say that, by asserting its aims through the tropes associated with New England, *CQ* represented a community that saw itself as less interested in and even more suspicious of professionalism than *MRPJ*.

At the same time, New England's greater emphasis on resisting professionalism serviced some of the needs of East Village dance. Artists whose reputation was unshaken by basing themselves in the pastoral regions north of New York, such as Paxton, Hay, Forti, Nelson, Stark Smith, and Lepkoff, brought to the East Village the significance of artistic integrity when they were programmed to teach and perform by Movement Research.[64] By connecting itself with New England Somatics, Movement Research, even as it promoted professionalism, seemed to retain a connection to earlier phases of experimentation and the aura of independence.[65] For New Yorkers, the symbolic integrity they extracted from their rural neighbors promised to fuel innovation in professional dance.

With the increasing institutionalization of New York Somatics in the 1980s onward, its New England equivalent claimed particular regimens for personal and artistic integrity. A rural setting configured itself as the proper context for developing Anatomical Releasing, CI, and other approaches that emphasized the exploration of anatomical function. For several years Nancy Topf, Marsha Paludan, and John Rolland, who with Fulkerson pioneered Anatomical Releasing, ran the Putney Workshop in rural Vermont along with Lepkoff, Stark Smith, and the CI dancer Christina Svane, encouraging students to work with the two forms together.[66] Dancers who went on to have a lifelong career based on their work with Somatics remember attending the Putney Workshop.[67] Meanwhile, Karczag, along with Giavenco and Webb, also retreated to Vermont to develop a pedagogy based on the teachings of Mabel Elsworth Todd's student André Bernard.

With its edict against technical elitism but connection to New York dance, New England provided a gateway for some dancers into lifelong careers. Lepkoff, Bill T. Jones and his partner Arnie Zane, Stephen Petronio, Randy Warshaw, Jennifer Miller, and many others first entered dance through CI, while dancers such as Diane Madden and Lisa Kraus exhibited the skills Brown sought for the work she began making in the late 1970s because they had accessed New England Somatics.[68] The seemingly more inclusive ethics of New England regimens also naturally contributed to New Yorkers' belief that in the regions north of the city they could reconnect with a sense of self not determined by professional demands. As the century progressed, dancers

chose either to invest in New York Somatics and develop virtuoso skills to execute what they saw as innovative choreography or to focus on what they felt
was greater personal and artistic integrity with New England Somatics. The
differences exhibited themselves in career choices, such as Madden's decision
to stay with Brown's company in various roles for the rest of her career, and
Karczag's decision to leave in the 1980s.[69]

It was through employment in isolated universities that some New
Englanders solved the problem of sustaining an artistic practice with relative independence from the professional field while also earning an income.
For example, Skinner and Anatomical Releasing both made their debut at
the University of Illinois at Urbana–Champaign, and Mary Fulkerson further developed Anatomical Releasing in her short-lived role from 1970 as the
head of the Rochester Collage dance program. Paxton also began teaching at
Bennington around the same time, and Lepkoff taught Somatics classes as
an adjunct professor at both Hampshire and Amherst later in the decade.[70]
By prioritizing research through New England Somatics, they reworked
Margaret H'Doubler's theory that the aims of dance education are in opposition to modern concert dance.[71] When artists took up residency in universities, they therefore instituted the idea of returning to the essence of art making
under the influence of progressive education principles that had survived in
Somatics.[72] Advocates of Somatics created teaching and research opportunities for independent artists to include students in the experimentation. The
artistic integrity, which rural living purportedly offered, thus linked itself with
the principle of independent reasoning associated with the Western academy
since the age of the Enlightenment. The connection between scholarship and
New England Somatics therefore reflects the idea that 1970s training affords
personal authenticity through modalities in which corporeality must be
approached with scientific objectivity. Dance students in higher education
found themselves configured as researchers of their own bodies.

Higher education also sustained the connection between New England and
New York Somatics because faculty explored ideas that they had either per-
sonally initiated in early 1960s New York dance or borrowed from that period. For example, Fulkerson configured Anatomical Releasing as inclusive,
extending to dance class the early 1960s idea of mixing trained and untrained
dancers.[73] She reframed the critique of virtuosity to connect artistic integrity
with the experiential analysis of the body. Dancers believed that their participation depended not on being skilled in a particular lexicon, but on their
willingness to explore imperatives of anatomical functioning.[74] Teaching artists also developed their choreography using students who were embodying
the new ideas.[75] Paxton, for example, met Lepkoff and David Woodberry as

Rochester College students, both of whom significantly contributed to the development of CI. Universities therefore offered alternative validation and the space for process-based work, but the results of research often found their way into the professional field.

Along with higher education, independent artists formed a quasi-autonomous network that sustained New England Somatics using festivals and residential workshops. Retaining the 1970s spirit of investigation, collaboration, and independence, the region functioned like an annex to New York. Artists who relocated to rural and provincial settings generated dance activity, of which students in the local university dance programs took advantage. Especially when the field was just establishing itself, adjunct faculty put their students in contact with the regional network beyond the institutions, which committed dancers went to some length to access. Madden recalls that she, Petronio, and Warshaw, all at Hampshire College, traveled nearly a hundred miles to Boston for a class with Lepkoff, but they also trained in BMC at Bainbridge Cohen's school in close-by Northampton.[76] Furthermore, New England festivals such as Jacob's Pillow bridged visiting dancers with New York; through concerts and classes, attendees accessed ideas that had not yet reached other regions.[77] Students also used the accessibility of New England Somatics to access New York dance, securing employment in a new brand of New York–based companies that required the skills developed in CI, Ideokinesis, or BMC. When they arrived in New York, some of these dancers took advantage of approaches explicitly geared toward company dancing.

The transnational community experienced New England Somatics in relation to New York. Across the network, the trope of returning to rural life resonated as one that would restore bodily and artistic integrity in training and aesthetics. Along with local dancers, foreign visitors to New York attended New England workshops, which they had learned about in CQ. They took the meaning attached to working in rural space beyond the throng of the city back to their local contexts, where teaching American artists also disseminated the ideas.[78] The symbolic significance of New England Somatics therefore accrued to artists throughout the network who employed choreographic strategies or pedagogies linked with the region.[79] Foreign dancers embodied the differences between New York and New England Somatics by learning to privilege investigation over presentation. For example, the British rural arts college Dartington, where Fulkerson headed a dance program beginning in 1972, positioned itself against London's modern dance–based training using New England Somatics.

The distinction between America's symbolic center for dance and its garden annex further imprinted itself on the transnational network through differences in the focus of *CQ* compared with *MRPJ*. The New York journal almost exclusively addressed dance within the city, while *CQ*, even though it primarily focused on American subscribers, enjoyed and referenced its transnational readership.[80] Consequently, dancers beyond the United States not familiar with the East Village milieu had no way of finding out about its collectivism, anticommercialism, and activism, instead meeting New York Somatics through successful choreographers. By contrast, they read about American dancers' critique of professionalism in *CQ*. Even though the CI community asserted its decentralization, New England housed *CQ* and was home to many of the pioneers, so the region provided a focus for CI. Therefore, in addition to claiming the critique of professionalism for the rural areas north of New York, *CQ* associated the duet form itself, as well as BMC and Authentic Movement, with New England. What is more, many of the large community gatherings chose remote settings, thereby further stressing the connection between the duet form and the land. Authentic Movement and BMC established their place in CI culture through dancers' interest in personal development, which made them a large clientele for the techniques. Writing about these approaches was published through Contact Editions, compared with a relative absence of articles about Klein Technique.[81] By using and contributing to the CI network, BMC and Authentic Movement enjoyed their association of independence from the professional circuit.

With its editorial policy of including diverse opinions, *CQ* privileged the liberal ideal of individual freedom of expression over any concerted criticism of institutionalization or commercialization in Somatics. Although the journal included expressions of discontent against the panoply of discourses that addressed ideas about the therapeutic benefits of dancing, and it hosted differing opinions about improvising, the potential for critique found itself engulfed by the generic backdrop of a community of individuals asserting their integrity. In this sense, *CQ* and New England Somatics, more generally, embodied American expansionist liberalism by stressing the importance for dancers of connecting with their authentic individual artistic perspectives beyond institutional and commercial structures. New England Somatics reflected the back-to-the-landers' aim to execute activism through a lifestyle more than anything else. The rural dance lifestyle saw its own version of this problem in the struggles over authenticity that ensued from its meanings. Furthermore, the American liberalism of New England Somatics met opposition in the body cultivated in Britain where individual authenticity was not enough to contest the domination of the conservative dance establishment.

British Somatics: The Political and Socially Signifying Body

British Somatics differed markedly from the New England focus on individual authenticity by framing itself collectively against a conservative dance establishment that had dismissed the first-wave American Somatics in the early 1970s. The dance establishment had rejected Somatics on the basis of a perceived lack of technical excellence and communicative accessibility. Two groups that welcomed Somatics, albeit with ambivalence, were Strider and X6, small but influential collectives of choreographers that formed in 1972 and 1976, respectively. By the 1980s, British Somatics had expanded sufficiently to begin to assert the independence of its socially conscious dance theater from American experimentation. Nevertheless, in all the different waves of their resistance, dancers embodied postwar American expansionist liberalism by reifying the natural body as a way to defy domestic protocols concerning aesthetics and expressive content while combating American dominance. By claiming freedom from technical standards and aesthetic formalism, they felt they "liberated" creative expression by addressing local concerns. Yet British Somatics ultimately revealed that liberalism underpinned its political overtones when they used the training as a means to artistic success within the very institutions that it had initially critiqued.

In the face of structural marginalization, British interest in Somatics first depended on connections with American artists. Strider, credited as Britain's first independent contemporary dance company, had declared their approach post-Cunningham in reaction against the ethos of the London School of Contemporary Dance (LSCD), the first modern dance training institution formed in 1969 that was based in Graham's pedagogy and aesthetic mission.[82] Strider initially staged "abstract" dance with Cunningham-like vocabulary, the innovation and technical proficiency of which the press embraced.[83] Yet when the collective drew on Somatics for experimentation, commentators turned on them, arguing that the caliber of the work was undermined.

Strider first encountered Somatics regimens through Fulkerson's Anatomical Releasing and improvisation training when they were in residence at Dartington College. There they discovered exciting new possibilities in Fulkerson's focus on anatomy.[84] To avoid isolation in her remote location, Fulkerson recycled the educational model she developed at Rochester, this time bringing Americans to Britain to teach New York and New England Somatics.[85] Like Strider, other young dancers seized on the regimens to forge new choreography as part of an unprecedented British independent dance

culture. The sources with which they associated Somatics therefore positioned America as a center for critical culture.

With institutional backing, and to celebrate the long-awaited accreditation of the dance program, Fulkerson also started the Dance at Dartington
festival in 1978. She brought together artists from America, Britain, and
other areas of Europe to perform, teach, and engage in debate. At a time
when many artists working with Somatics were isolated with few resources,
Dartington became a crucial hub for the development of the transnational
community. Because the majority of the festival's teachers and performers
were American, and the British establishment remained so hostile, the
college appeared to be an outpost developing New York experimental culture. For example, the first festival offered classes taught by Topf, Paxton,
Paludan, and Fulkerson herself. All the teachers also performed along with
another of Fulkerson's colleagues from Illinois, Nancy Udow. Dartington
also hosted Paxton as a resident teacher from 1974 to 1978.[86] The college
thus established itself as a foothold for disseminating the regimens in and
beyond Britain by virtue of American artists to whom Fulkerson offered
vital opportunities to develop their work.

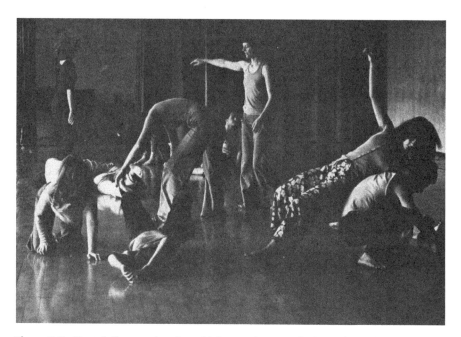

Figure 2.3. Mary Fulkerson dancing with her students as she is teaching class at
Dartington, 1982. Fulkerson is standing center, right arm raised.
Photograph by Brian Haslem. © Arts Archive (Council of Europe).

Faced with suspicion from the British establishment about the value of Somatics, Fulkerson and her colleagues used the liberal ideal of individual creative freedom to institutionalize the training. This overcame the discrepancy between Somatics and establishment protocols on British concert dance by framing the pedagogy as developing the compositional artistry of each dancer instead of their performance ability. The Council for National Academic Accreditation rejected Dartington's first application, and the changes that were subsequently made reveal how Somatics negotiated the British establishment.[87] The second and successful application focused on how students were said to be interrogating movement rather than mastering an existing vocabulary. It also concealed Fulkerson's interest in mundane gesture and untrained dancers.[88] Nonetheless, in contrast with other institutions, Dartington relieved incoming students of the requirement of previous training.[89] The emphasis on individual creativity in Somatics appealed to artists wanting to work outside of large companies, and at the time Fulkerson's institutional foothold was an oasis when Britain offered few funding or other opportunities for concert dance outside of ballet and two modern companies. Stephanie Jordan documents how independent choreographers and dancers faced "severe problems of funding [in] the mid-1970s."[90] Many artists thus shared Fulkerson's marginalization at the hands of the establishment and drew creative and moral resources from her and the other Americans teaching at Dartington and its festival. They aligned themselves with Somatics based in their sense of shared marginalization. X6 specifically used the training to embody the group's feminist principles even though they deplored what they saw as the apolitical nature of New York choreography in general, during the period when artists such as Brown were rapidly being embraced by the British press and theaters.

In 1976, with X6's declaration of its basis in a feminist orientation, London was more directly confronted by artists challenging the establishment on administrative, ideological, and aesthetic levels.[91] Using Somatics, the collective critiqued sexist ideals of gender in training, which they perceived to be integral to the virtuosity demanded by the establishment. X6 felt that the natural female body was erased by balletic aesthetics, which enforced a hierarchy putting women in competition to become passive tools for male choreographers. To foreground dancers' health and autonomy in response, they invested in the idea of working with natural functional imperatives of the body.[92] They also critiqued conventional masculinity, using what they saw as the irrelevance of gender in CI to cut through social difference by focusing on anatomical structure. Along with other dancers, X6 developed an artistic culture they called "New Dance." The first generation of Fulkerson's graduates began teaching, taking classes, and presenting work in a loose London network in which X6 was pivotal.[93]

X6's problem with what they saw as apolitical abstraction created tension in New Dance concerning what constituted British Somatics. Although they shared the periphery with Fulkerson, X6 perceived American Somatics as contributing to aesthetics that were eventually endorsed, primarily through the work of Richard Alston, by the dance establishment. The initial enthusiasm for Strider's early Cunningham-like work probably built on the press's perception that Cunningham's choreography constituted a combination of innovation and technical excellence. By the late 1970s, Strider's founding member, Richard Alston, was similarly embraced by the establishment when he choreographed for large companies and began using classical aesthetics including pointe work.[94] Alston credited Fulkerson as key to his artistic development, so for artists staging political themes, it seemed that Somatics could support dance of which they were highly critical.[95] In the late 1970s and early 1980s, however, British programmers favored New York dance rich in complex steps and devoid of explicit themes.[96] When the Dance Umbrella festival did showcase New Dance, it chose British artists such as Rosemary Butcher and Maedée Duprès, who identified with New York formalism and avoided social commentary.[97] Although initially an X6 member, Duprès's choreography contrasted with her colleagues Fergus Early, Jacky Lansley, Emilyn Claid, and Mary Prestidge. The establishment ignored or vilified the rest of the collective who, with performance art strategies rather than formal dance innovation, staged explicitly political content.[98]

As a result of the tensions in New Dance, a bifurcation occurred between American formalism and British political dance. The reticence of the state to fund any independent British ventures provided a continuing basis for an uneasy alliance. However, the press exacerbated the association of "formalism" with America in the early 1980s and positioned Brits working in a comparable manner as derivative.[99] X6 publicly tracked and critiqued funding and programming, identifying patterns of privilege. In the late 1970s it appeared that classicism met establishment protocols, followed by large modern companies and New York formalism, while third in line was formalist British dance, and explicitly political work was given the lowest priority for funding and programming.[100] This naturally put strain on the New Dance community.

Some choreographers associated with X6 critiqued British choreographers who used the regimens for formal innovation.[101] Claid, for example, insisted on the political redundancy of creating new vocabulary because, she argued, dance must directly address existing social structures and aesthetic traditions. Claid held that British contemporary dance needed structural change rather than innovation. To achieve gender critique, she deconstructed classical narrative, which perhaps also explains her repurposing rather than rejection of ballet. She and her colleagues integrated Somatics to minimize physical stress in an anticompetitive and antihierarchical culture where students exchanged ideas with their teachers and each other.[102] Yet some other artists, such as Karczag, felt they could better stage gender critique using casual or quotidian vocabulary that rejected the classical idiom. Karczag, however, who immigrated to Britain from Australia to join the London Festival Ballet and then left to join Strider, appeared to have engaged in the very innovation against which Claid railed.[103]

Despite a divide between New Dance artists over the significance of American choreography, they continued to capitalize on New York's significance as the center of modern dance to fight for their own visibility and harvest ideas through exchange with visiting artists. For example, the dancers who aligned themselves with Brown when the press attacked *Glacial Decoy* insisted that had critics followed comparable developments in the British New Dance movement, they would not have been so ill informed about what constitutes technical virtuosity. Even so, while none of the independent commentators agreed with the mainstream press about the lack of technical proficiency in Brown's work, some did deplore *Glacial Decoy* for being apolitical.[104] So even though dancers were drawn together against the establishment, structural exclusion was not enough to gloss their differences.

However, the tolerance of contradictions between artists who took inspiration from choreographers like Brown and those who saw her as failing to address the most important concerns gave British Somatics its strength. The editorial policy of *New Dance Magazine* (*NDM*), which X6 began in 1977, allowed for a unifying platform between the divided interests of independent artists. *NDM* aimed to remedy what its editors saw as a critical vacuum because of the grip of classical ideals and Graham technique on British dance.[105] Like its transatlantic counterparts, *NDM* registered independent classes, but its writers also focused on politics and inequality to critique dance conservatism before either *CQ* or *MRPJ* addressed these issues with any consistency.[106] A rich if fraught late 1970s and early 1980s New Dance culture emerged because artists such as Laurie Booth, Rosemary Butcher, Miranda Tufnell, Dennis Greenwood, Julyen Hamilton, and Kirstie Simson, who were fascinated by the new movement possibilities of Somatics, shared spaces with the X6 collective, and they all saw each other's work.

Ultimately, however, to establish independence, British artists constructed a national contemporary dance identity, distancing themselves from New York through their staging of social themes. Politicized choreography asserted itself as uniquely British, not least because formalism was associated with America. What is more, those invested in social themes argued that formalism was theoretically flawed, which exacerbated the identification of independent dancers with distinct national tendencies. Artists not working with explicit themes consequently aligned themselves with New York, or were defined as such by default, and interdisciplinary social critique claimed itself as a peculiarly British aesthetic.[107] Jordan reports that, rather than look to New York, X6 artists "decided that, as British artists, they would build directly from their experience in Britain."[108]

A new generation of dancers in the 1980s somewhat resolved the tensions with the emergence of British "Dance Theatre."[109] Companies such as DV8 Physical Theatre choreographed social themes using new vocabulary informed by Somatics, which benefited from the experiments undertaken in the 1970s. In what many Brits referred to as the "dance boom" after the paucity of resources in the previous decade, new young artists secured state funding, played in established theaters, and received sympathetic press. Changes at the Dartington festival contributed to this cultural shift, both by increasing the number of British New Dance artists and teachers that it programmed relative to Americans and by displacing its early culture of exchange and experimentation and becoming an alternative national showcase. The changes demonstrate how British nationalism rose as collective ideals diminished.

In Thatcher's entrepreneurial culture, artists constructed unique signatures to represent feminist and queer subjects that, while opposing the government's conservative cultural agenda, nevertheless rode upon its rhetoric about the value of individual gain. Furthermore, despite the choreography's progressive overtures, artists performed to largely white middle-class audiences. Claid, for example, points out that "while white artists were rejecting conventional European aesthetics of identity, black British dance artists were seeking an identifiable presence," which created "a paradox between subjectivity and in/visibility."[110] For Claid, this meant that "as black and white dance artists we worked in parallel with each other but not together."[111] Even community dance, which also emerged out of the political concerns of the 1970s, failed to exceed the tenets of liberalism by extending a state agenda. Artists using Somatics choreographed within working-class and minority communities, hoping to make contemporary dance accessible to people that otherwise would not have accessed the art. However, rather than critique inequality, they therefore served as artistic missionaries for bourgeois values.[112]

The initial struggle for British Somatics to establish itself contributed to the development of the transnational network while reasserting New York's dominance. With evangelical zeal, artists and educators promoted Somatics and, through Dance at Dartington, established an expansionist agenda for British Somatics that rivaled its corollaries from New York and New England. At the college country manor, established artists and unknowns danced, ate, and lived together, while the classes welcomed students of all experience levels. Artists struggling to gain critical recognition in their native contexts garnered support from the festival's transnational scope based on New York's cultural capital, because key American figures added importance to the festival. Meanwhile, those who were isolated at home felt they were re-establishing links with New York, which for Dutch and Australian dancers, for example, positioned Dartington as a more accessible way to access New York Somatics. Similarly, Australians could more easily study and work in Britain than in America, and this impact is visible, as we will see, in the Australian journal *Writings on Dance*.

By the 1990s, British and New York Somatics mirrored each other. Like Movement Research, Chisenhale Dance Space (CDS), the daughter of X6, focused on the exploration rather than production of dance, and continued to battle with the establishment, while Independent Dance (ID) offered daily professional Somatics classes and workshops in a more formal vein. Politics and professionalism were never neatly divided between the two organizations, but dancers using Somatics for technical excellence could attend ID classes, while those pursuing an exploratory approach would be more likely to use CDS.[113] The divergence exhibited itself in the techniques and artists associated with the different contexts; for example, ID ran a daily technique class that applied ideas from various Somatics regimens to set movement. Dancers associated with successful British choreography often taught ID's regular training, but the organization also employed Americans who danced with large companies and used Klein Technique.[114] Meanwhile, rather than regular classes, CDS tended to offer workshops that combined training and exploration based on the approach of individual artists.[115]

London, however, exhibited an important difference from New York in that British artists not focusing on either politics or formalism slipped between the cracks. New England Somatics supported an improvisation scene in New York through the East Village, while London never established such a context. *NDM* had provided a discursive context for Brits improvising with Somatics, but following its collapse in 1986, such artists became increasingly marginalized. Nonetheless, the growth of equivalencies between New York and London exhibited the impact of commercialism and institutionalization in the 1980s and 1990s. The two cities found themselves linked by transnational dance culture, to which the independent Somatics network had contributed but now played a secondary role. The British establishment reconstructed itself in the dance boom, imposing new aesthetic and technical protocols for Dance Theatre. Fulkerson marked this sea change when, in 1988, she moved from Dartington to Holland in search of new resources to cultivate independent transnational Somatics.

Dutch Somatics: The Body in Flux

Unlike Britain, Dutch Somatics found itself almost exclusively housed in higher education, which made it possible for proponents, in their implementation of the regimens, to largely avoid the impact of dance critics' opinions or the programming policies of concert houses. Instead, education based on the regimens survived through ties with the transnational network. By sidestepping what was endorsed by theaters and critics, proponents working in state conservatories constructed a body "in flux," framing dance training as individual investigation for which outcomes cannot be anticipated. In its renouncing of identifiable aesthetics, Dutch Somatics nonetheless emphasized liberalism by configuring the natural body as a site at which the dissident individual artist oversteps existing social structures.

In the first of two phases of development beginning in the early 1970s, Pauline De Groot helped to create the first modern dance program in Amsterdam's state arts conservatory (Amsterdamse Hogeschool voor de Kunsten or AHK). Based on the training to which Erick Hawkins had introduced her as his company member, De Groot consolidated a process-based pedagogy in opposition with classical and modern dance. Along with other artists trained in the regimens and support from those interested in the new training, the approach that De Groot introduced ultimately achieved dominance within the institution. The program found itself at odds with other Dutch professional dancers, however, when they withdrew from the institution because they were opposed to its experimental pedagogy and aesthetics.[116] Employing Americans such as Trude Cone, who trained in Lulu Sweigard's interpretation of Mabel Elsworth Todd's work at Julliard, and later John Rolland, the program saw itself as part of an international milieu in which its pedagogy and aesthetics were embraced.

A second late 1980s expansionist phase followed the establishing of a new AHK program based on Graham and Cunningham techniques, which resulted in the reformation of the Somatics-based department as the School voor Nieuwe Dansontwikkeling (SNDO, or School for New Dance Development). The state conservatory in Arnhem (De Hogeschool voor de Kunsten Arnhem, or HKA) simultaneously established its own Somatics-based program, initially known as the Centrum voor Nieuwe Dansontwikkeling (CNDO, or Center for New Dance Development). The Arnhem school, ultimately called the European Dance Development Center (EDDC), further extended its program to the Tanzwerkplatz in Dusseldorf, Germany, and pursued unfulfilled plans for a program in Lisbon, Portugal. Through temporary foreign teachers that the schools employed from beyond the Netherlands, Dutch Somatics established a codependent relationship with the rest of the transnational network. Visitors brought pedagogic and creative resources while benefiting from exchange and employment at the institutions that became pivotal to the transnational community. Because of its location within education, Somatics-trained dancers did not create independent organizations because they coalesced and supported each other within the schools. Local artists did not therefore produce a publication but instead focused on independent contexts with which they could be in contact as they emerged across multiple Anglophone sites.[117]

Recycling the idea that dancers were training as creative rather than interpretive artists, Dutch Somatics perhaps emphasized individuality more than any other transnational hub. Students investigated kinetic possibility by cultivating kinesthetic awareness, working with pedestrian movement, and using lower muscle tone than in classical and modern training. First instituted in her independent Amsterdam studio, De Groot developed her pedagogy in relative isolation. Her classes resembled Anatomical Releasing and betrayed ideas common in the work being undertaken by Brown, Forti, Paxton, and Fulkerson, including feeling the influences of Ideokinesis and H'Doubler through Halprin.[118] De Groot initiated a Dutch equivalent on the basis that training could engender experimentation as the very basis of a contemporary dancing body.

In a further correlation with Britain, American expansionism impacted Dutch Somatics in a way that caused domestic conflict. Along with others who had trained and performed in American modern dance, the new AHK program invited De Groot to contribute to its formation. Yet unlike her colleagues, De Groot rejected the idea that modern dance should underpin the training.[119] Initially, the moderns and De Groot allied with each other against teachers who wanted all students to have a classical ballet foundation.[120] When a purely modern program established itself in 1976, however, Somatics revealed its incompatibility with Graham technique. The balletomanes and moderns felt Somatics would undermine dancers' professionalism. Classical teachers argued students would lack extension and elevation, and Graham teachers insisted that the strength they were cultivating ran counter to the "softness" of Somatics.[121] Meanwhile, De Groot believed students would have

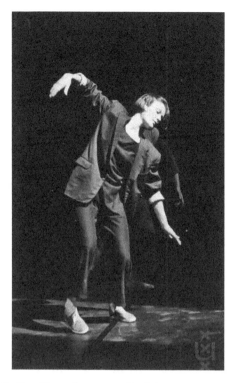

Figure 2.4. Pauline De Groot in performance. No date.
Photograph by Maarten Brinkgreve. Collectie TIN.

to unlearn modern and classical technique to cultivate sensory awareness, which was essential to integrating creative exploration in training.[122] Modern dance at the AHK therefore inherited a conflict within the artistic traditions they imported from America.

The Netherlands amplified the incompatibilities that New York dance established that had also caused conflict in Britain because De Groot instituted Somatics in the Netherlands' cultural capital. This magnified its conflict with Graham and Cunningham technique because all the approaches were arguing at the same time for their superiority as a means to cultivate a national modern dance. De Groot's belief in the opposition between the individual and authoritarianism convinced her of the incompatibility of modern dance and Somatics. She argued that the imposition of modern vocabulary instituted a mindless physical regimen, which she had slowly discarded as a Hawkins dancer. Working with Mabel Elsworth Todd's student André Bernard at Hawkins's behest, De Groot recalls an agonizing "unlearning process": letting go of the skills she developed through arduous labor in Graham and ballet training. Yet she felt "her life and meaning" were consequently allowed to "stream through her," and that was what De Groot sought for her students. Although she believed in an eclectic training, something she also inherited from Hawkins, De Groot resisted integration with the modern techniques because she believed that to integrate creativity with daily movement practice, the authoritarianism in classical and modern training must be replaced by Somatics.[123] Moreover, the modern teachers characterized their techniques as hard against hers as soft, which for De Groot reduced all of her philosophy and politics to a question of muscle tension. Yet despite the misinterpretation to which she felt she was subject and her high ideals for her students, with her insistence upon the importance of individual creative freedom, De Groot brought with her to the AHK a model of training that embodied postwar American liberalism.

The directorate initially resolved the diversity of opinions about training held by faculty with a semiautonomous structure that reflected a broader national culture of mediating between differences through what is known as pillarization. Since the beginning of the twentieth century, the Netherlands had negotiated social, political, and religious differences by establishing distinct social spheres in Catholic, Protestant, socialist, and liberal "pillars." While pillarization diminished after the 1960s, unprecedented postwar state funding of pillared organizations left a lasting impact and, at its height, highly distinct pillars or spheres, such as the financial, political, educational, entertainment, health, community, and labor. Late twentieth-century immigrants even formed their own pillars. Commentators attribute to the system both Dutch tolerance toward social diversity and a lack of integration and dialog between different groups that could result, for example, in racism.[124] Although De Groot was initially allowed to develop her ideas as a pillar, enjoying relative autonomy compared with Fulkerson's struggle to establish academic accreditation in Britain, the AHK eventually required De Groot's students to train in ballet and modern dance, which forced the teachers into antagonistic dialog with each other. Students also struggled with the different training, which only exacerbated the tension.[125]

After ongoing conflict with modern dance throughout the 1970s, Somatics established its dominance at the AHK by the end of the decade. The institution employed two key figures to resolve the differences between faculty, but both of the arbiters found themselves convinced by what they saw as the more progressive solution to training that De Groot offered. Aat Hougée became a proponent of Somatics after he began administrating the quasi-autonomous relationship of De Groot's studio to the AHK.[126] Her artistic philosophy dovetailed with his political background reflecting a broader antiauthoritarian

Dutch cultural zeitgeist of which the 1960s countercultural Provo movement was indicative. The Provos used nonviolence and absurd humor to create social change, taking their inspiration from anarchism, Dadaism, the German philosopher Herbert Marcuse, and the Marquis de Sade, all of which they exhibited through performance arts pranks intended to fool and frustrate government agencies.[127] In this milieu, Hougée developed a taste for antiauthoritarian client-centered learning through participation in a 1960s mental health treatment reform movement.[128] Hougée's background resonated with De Groot's philosophy, and she found that her ideas also paralleled the Provos' anarchic use of music, poetry, and performance as a strategy of protest.[129]

Hougée and De Groot eventually took up directorship of the school along with the Graham teacher Bart Stuyf, who posed no serious opposition to their approach.[130] When Cone and Rolland joined the faculty, they extended the range of Somatics classes on offer. Antagonism persisted with modern teachers, however, and the AHK replaced De Groot with Jaap Flier when De Groot rescinded her leadership. Flier, as a Dutch ballet star who also trained in and performed modern dance, promised to bring resolve because of his background in technique, esteemed position in Dutch dance, and international sophistication, which the administration thought would position him to mediate between the artistic differences. But as with Hougée, the individual creativity and antiauthoritarianism of Somatics convinced Flier of its value and pre-eminence. As someone who had directed and choreographed large companies based on classical and modern training, which he had also taught, Flier sought a pedagogy with a "goal that one can share . . . and give each other information . . . [to take] it away for me from being a student-teacher situation."[131] The remaining modern teachers left by the early 1980s, paving the way for Somatics to crystallize based on the renouncing of any predetermined vocabulary, and the faculty consolidated their ethos by framing the school as a laboratory.

The Dutch schools worked with a great volume of visiting artists to emphasize the cultivation of individual artistic processes rather than the emulation of a style. By employing teaching artists who were often not well supported by their domestic establishments, Hougée, for example, insisted that the approaches taught at the school were independent of the professional demand for success.[132] New England artists such as Forti, Paxton, Lepkoff, and Nelson brought pedagogy to the school based on their solo improvisational practices that emphasized exploration as opposed to commercial success. Meanwhile, with their recalcitrant dancing bodies, East Village artists contributed a critique of 1970s aesthetics at a time when the new complex vocabulary seen on large concert stages seemed to have claimed Somatics for its own. Dutch education therefore reasserted the dissidence of the regimens when the natural body seemed to be losing its critical potential.[133] EDDC solidified its antiprofessionalist position by presenting itself to prospective students as a program that would equip them to work in marginal rather than mainstream dance.[134]

Housed within the laboratory frame of the schools, permanent faculty also intensified their own explorations of how individual creativity could be developed. For example, Karczag wanted students to oppose the idea of the dancer as a tool for the choreographer by resisting recognizable vocabulary. Her pedagogy extended from her solo improvising rather than her history as a company dancer and aimed at movement that flouted aesthetic traditions.[135] Karczag, who was on the permanent faculty from the late 1980s, looked to teaching artists such as Paxton and combined Ideokinesis, CI, tai chi, and Alexander Technique, cultivating what she saw as an expanded kinetic form to provide students with physical and artistic space to move.[136] Her colleague, Tony Thatcher, sought unanticipated outcomes by challenging the premise that students knew what it was that they wanted to do as a dancer or to see as a choreographer.[137] Like Karczag, he was influenced by Alexander Technique and encouraged students to consider that being or feeling "wrong" could broaden their creative possibility.[138] Faculty theorized individuality in opposition to existing aesthetics and company structures; they therefore aimed to engender creative potential through training, rather than preparing the students for employment in existing companies.

Students within the various manifestations of higher education within the Netherlands sometimes rejected the faculty's ideas about experimentation. All the same, they did so through a discourse of discovering a personal aesthetic rather than emulating an established form. Those who were not cognizant of the context or history against which their teachers were reacting experienced the training as an imposition of aesthetics in exactly the way that faculty wanted to avoid. For example, some students felt under pressure to discard what appeared to be control or precision in their dancing because it challenged the aesthetics through which the teachers were affirming their ideology.[139] Consequently, through the institutionalization of resistance toward the reproduction of an established form, a dominant aesthetic emerged, one that manifested physical looseness and unpredictability from one movement choice to the next.[140] To critique the training they received, students also used the idea of personal development and healing that was integral to the rhetoric in the regimens. For example, they demanded access to psychotherapy, arguing that education relies on the interrogation of self and therefore arouses emotional confusion, and they campaigned for resources to address this.[141]

Thus, regardless of whether they accepted the faculty's aesthetics, those who pursued their dance education in Dutch Somatics embodied the ethics of individuality.[142]

In a manner similar to the way that professionalism haunted New England Somatics, Dutch educators created a specter out of reproducing existing form through their emphasis on escaping any recognizable vocabulary. They also disagreed with each other about how to cultivate individuality, which reflected the growing concern about the development of a Somatics style in Dutch education and further afield in the other transnational hubs that fed the schools. For example, SNDO teacher Gonnie Hegen, who trained at the institution in the 1980s, argued that Somatics did not cultivate individuality because students embodied images that, while not related to the "self," stood in for personal authenticity. Much like Cone's insistence that American experimental aesthetics had stood for individuality at SNDO, Hegen launched a valuable critique of Somatics. Yet also like Cone, rather than exposing the fallacy of the pedagogy itself—that of training students to achieve individual artistic authenticity—she introduced her own pedagogy that sustained the liberal ideology of creative freedom. Hegen taught structures that demanded rapid change in action to avert preconceived movement ideas, which she felt restored uniqueness. However, accelerated redirection simply replaced the looseness, internal focus, and unpredictability of movement choice that had previously signified individuality.[143] Meanwhile, student allegiances that developed at CNDO/EDDC in Arnhem exhibited similar struggle with the issue of how to achieve individuality while avoiding the reproduction of a recognizable vocabulary. For example, some students affiliated with Karczag used anatomical imagery and emphasized the physical body as a mystical source of untapped creative resources, while others associated themselves with Fulkerson, who insisted upon the value of psychological and symbolic images as a way to move beyond the limits of focusing on physicality. By reflecting a broader transnational concern about the crystallization of Somatics style as the century progressed, the schools betrayed the way in which they enjoyed less independence from professional dance than they might have liked to think.

SNDO and CNDO/EDDC directors interpreted their alienation from domestic dance differently. Hougée strengthened the connection between New York and the Arnhem school, fostering a belief that a domestic lack of appreciation for his mission was a sign of parochialism. De Groot supported Hougée because, since the early 1970s, she had felt her choreography was more warmly embraced abroad.[144] But Cone believed that solipsistic dances had alienated Dutch audiences, because students were immersed in research and unconcerned with communication.[145] Indeed, Hougée prioritized research over reaching audiences with his belief that the artist is a necessary generator of novel cultural language, a role that he felt cultural centers inhibited because innovation would get appropriated through the professional demand for success.[146] By pitting education against domestic dance, he neglected consideration of the context in which pedagogy might be located and instead argued that employment at the schools also supported the independence of transnational artists from their domestic professional contexts.

The student population reflected the increasingly transnational focus of Dutch Somatics. During the 1970s, substantial numbers of Dutch students attended the Amsterdam school, yet their numbers dwindled with the loss of domestic support. At the same time, the presence of key transnational figures for Somatics ignited foreign interest. Fulkerson's codirectorship strengthened the transnational scope of SNDO, and subsequently CNDO/EDDC, because of her previous pivotal role through Dartington in the network between hubs in Britain, American, and Australia.[147] Foreign students thus heard about the school by word of mouth and through publications circulating in the hubs.[148] They flocked to Holland to work with a range of experimental dancers in an approach to training unrivaled beyond the Netherlands. Hence, Dutch Somatics increasingly depended on foreigners for its ongoing development.

SNDO and CNDO/EDDC replaced Dartington as the European juncture for transnational exchange when the Dartington festival ceased and Fulkerson moved to the Netherlands.[149] British Somatics subsequently integrated into domestic dance, diminishing its connections to the transnational community, except for those artists whose work exceeded establishment protocols and who relied on overseas opportunities to find significance for their work largely because they focused on process.[150] Meanwhile, foreign artists working in Holland misrecognized the success of Dutch Somatics as resulting from the Netherlands' more laissez-faire culture as compared with Anglophone contexts. In fact, the history of pillarization enabled dance education and its professional corollary to exist alongside each other in relative noncommunication, and rather than being viewed domestically as a basis for tolerance, Dutch progressives challenged domestic cultural partition in the 1960s on the basis that it restricted choice through religious and other affiliations, even to the point of employment opportunities.[151] To some degree, we can understand the eventual domination that Somatics achieved at the AHK as a product of this social shift, because with its rhetoric of individual choice, the training dovetailed with the wider challenge to pillarization. Yet, by positioning itself as the only training within which dancers could make individual choices, Dutch Somatics recycled America's expansionism in which the opportunity for freedom of expression in various global contexts supposedly depends on American cultural, economic, and military domination. Dancers from contexts that still marginalized the approach experienced Somatics discipline as resulting from a doctrine of tolerance that included such policies as both sexes changing into their dance clothes together right next to the director's office. Because they equated freedom of expression with tolerance, they failed to detect the inability of modern and Somatics teachers to collaborate and the expansionist underpinnings of the training.

Australian Somatics: The New Frontier

Like its Dutch equivalent, Australian Somatics sought to expand and enrich local approaches to training and composition through participation in a transnational context; however, practitioners from Australia framed their practice as part of a newly invigorated dedication to experimentation within the arts, supported, in part, by the establishment in 1967 of the Australia Council (later the Australian Arts Council). Although their approach came from abroad, dancers believed that renewable originality in the regimens meant that Somatics could nurture an independent Australian voice and bring new and important insights to the entire dance community, regardless of their prior training. Dancers worked with experimental musicians and theater practitioners in a budding avant-garde that also introduced new approaches to composition.

After participating in American and British contemporary dance, a handful of Australians brought ideas back home, including Nanette Hassall and Russell Dumas, who formed the Sydney-based collective Dance Exchange in 1976. They were joined by Karczag later that year.[152] As well as performing with major ballet and contemporary companies in New York and London, the three danced with London's Strider earlier in the decade and employed a similar approach once they returned to Sydney.[153] Hassall and Karczag introduced Anatomical Releasing and improvisatory procedures they had encountered with Fulkerson, and Hassall also used the aleatory methods she learned as a Cunningham dancer, while Dumas developed the movement puzzles he absorbed from working with Brown, Twyla Tharp, and Sara Rudner. Classes offered at Dance Exchange also frequently included approaches taken from CI. Together, Somatics and "pure movement" seemed to be specific to no culture but offer unique artistic expression through a broadened range of aesthetic options, sourced from movement capacity and integral to human physiology.

Dance Exchange repurposed Fulkerson's missionary narrative and the rhetoric that New Dance was helping isolated regional British and European artists achieve liberation. The ways that Australians worked to establish alternative aesthetic choices also paralleled the advocacy that Hougée exerted for Somatics within the Dutch domestic scene. Like British artists, the Australians rejected establishment aesthetics, although they worked with funding agencies and critics to bring awareness of the new dance practices to the public. Unique to 1970s Somatics, the Australian dancers embodied the idea evident in early American modern dance of being a new frontier of Western culture.

Dancers working with Somatics largely aspired to be part of an international Anglophone network, preferring to see themselves as connecting with a global cutting edge, and they looked to the other transnational centers for creative resources. For example, Dance Exchange seemed like the new frontier of a transnational project because they employed strategies they learned witnessing the downtown dance scene in New York and working in Britain with Strider. Similar to the Judson artists and to Strider, they worked in cheap makeshift venues educating their audiences with workshops connected to their concerts.[154] The dancers also replicated the antihierarchal company structures in New York and London; they shared organizational roles, danced in each other's choreography, and hosted work by artists with whom they shared values.[155] At the same time, by configuring themselves as a new frontier of experimental art, they embodied Western cultural expansionism.

With the cultural power that the avant-garde began to accrue, Australian Somatics enjoyed a substantially different reception from its British equivalent. Some Australian dance critics promoted Dance Exchange as the new artistic frontier. They agreed with the collective that balletic ideals were vestiges of colonial conservatism, and therefore sympathized with the use of Somatics. Unlike Strider, whose initial success came before working with the regimens and who were then denounced once they incorporated it, the members of Dance Exchange already had a history with the training when they arrived in Australia, so Somatics always infused their choreography and performance.[156] While Strider lost its funding when the company began working with Fulkerson, Dance Exchange, in a context of warm press support, rapidly received funding from the Theatre Board of the Australian Council with their use of Somatics.[157]

Differences in the press representation of Strider and Dance Exchange also reveal why the idea of a new frontier worked so well. Even when the critics supported the British collective prior to their work with Fulkerson, writers saw themselves as arbiters of established taste, judging a young company's

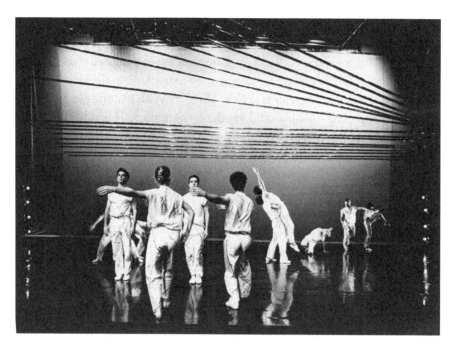

Figure 2.5. *Openweave,* choreographed by Nanette Hassall and created for the Australian Dance Theatre (ADT). Set and costume design: Mary Moore Music: Robert Lloyd. Performed at the Playhouse—Adelaide Festival Centre, March 1987. Photograph by David Wilson.

potential to fulfill self-evident aesthetic criteria.[158] By contrast, assuming there was broad unfamiliarity with modern dance, Australian critics educated their readership about Dance Exchange.[159] Hassall and Dumas asserted that Dance Exchange was taking risks and exploring the new rather than sustaining tradition.[160] Dumas argued that because Australia tended to emulate European culture to achieve sophistication, its modern choreography was a diluted European copy of American ideas. Hassall matched his rhetoric by distinguishing Dance Exchange from Australian modern ballet. She acknowledged its influence but also characterized it as committed to tradition rather than risk.[161] Critics explained to their readers that Dance Exchange differed from other companies with their use of ease as opposed to tension, and explained that the "release" method provides a greater breadth of vocabulary.[162]

Despite the effort to establish the Australian character of Dance Exchange's practice, the press and dancers continued to validate the company's value by linking it to an international context. Writers emphasized the collective's New York and London credentials, imbuing them with sophistication and providing evidence for the value of their risk-taking. The artists appeared to have forfeited their international careers to develop domestic dance. For example, writing about a Dance Exchange 1977 residency at RMIT, Melbourne's university of design and technology, Donna Greaves admitted that it "might seem at first an unusual place for people used to working in the artistically sophisticated circles of London and New York."[163] With histories in what were seen as world-class classical and modern companies, Hassall and Dumas seemed to have the ability to distinguish between real innovation and the emulation of outdated traditions or watered-down modernism. Dance Exchange therefore positioned itself as at the vanguard of a new national dance culture.

In subsequent years, after Karczag had left Australia, Hassall and Dumas nurtured a new generation, encouraging them to make their own work and introducing them to overseas artists.[164] In 1983, Hassall set up her Melbourne-based company and production house Dance Works through which many dancers and choreographers were nurtured. Artists such as Becky Hilton and Lucy Guerin worked as part of Dance Works and subsequently with Dumas, who in turn introduced them, along with Ros Warby, to Sara Rudner on state-funded trips to New York. Dumas also brought artists such as Lisa Nelson to Australia to give workshops.[165] Hassall and her students also quickly established Somatics in educational institutions, reaching a new generation with an Anatomical Releasing approach taught in an almost identical manner in other contexts.[166] Elizabeth Dempster, who had participated in British New Dance, worked with Hassall and went on to teach Somatics elsewhere in Australia.[167] New students therefore learned of the transnational network from their teachers, and through *CQ* and *NDM*, which circulated in institutional settings.

The domestic publication *Writings on Dance*, a legacy of Dance Exchange's endeavors, evidenced the emphasis on the transnational network and the trope of Australia being a new frontier for Somatics.[168] Despite government and press support for Dance Exchange, *Writings on Dance* saw isolation as a key domestic problem. For example, in a report on a "small dance companies" conference in the 1987 issue, coeditor Sally Gardner betrays the feeling that the consolidation of an independent dance scene remained beyond Australia's reach. She insisted that dancers and choreographers need a critical framework to be able to talk to each other.[169] The journal therefore attempted to resolve the problem by addressing what its other coeditor, Dempster, observed as the "absence of a critical space for dance . . . in Melbourne [and] Australia."[170] *Writings on Dance* consequently differed from its foreign equivalents by philosophically interrogating artists' practice and aiming to educate dancers about Somatics.[171] For example, the first issue in 1985 boasts an extensive article in which Ann Thompson aims to "consider . . . ideokinesis and related image processes within the current, social, economic and political context."[172] She provides a detailed description of Mabel Elsworth Todd's pedagogy and its application for dancers through, for example, "release technique," but also considers how the approach is liberatory for women by framing the ideas about image developed in John Berger's *Ways of Seeing*.[173] Although the journal differed from *NDM*, its ongoing interest in feminism betrays strong links between British and Australian artists and the recycling of X6's strategy of aiming to deal with isolation and lack of resources by nurturing critical perspectives to establish a robust independent context.[174] The depth and rigor with which writers addressed various issues in *Writings on Dance* reflect an artistic milieu that saw itself as pioneering with Somatics into uncharted territory.

The new excitement around dance can be seen, in retrospect, to have participated in a broader 1970s Australian cultural independence movement in which practitioners from various fields aimed to achieve a national movement that connected to the cutting-edge arts that were circulating between major Western hubs such as New York and London. From this perspective, dancers formed part of a pioneer narrative in which postcolonial cultural independence was achieved by breaking new ground for the international venture of contemporary dance. By importing Somatics, they claimed to source bodily truths with which local dance could be liberated from the lasting cultural influence of British colonialism. To assert their experimentalism, dancers configured the natural body as a source from which a distinctly Australian voice could be cultivated that exceeded domestic limitations to speak to international concerns. The Australian experience thus highlights the role of internationalism and authenticity in the use of the regimens.

Throughout the period of its growth, Somatics formed part of a progressive turn, exhibited first in legal changes that rejected outdated colonial logic. Indigenous Australians achieved full citizenship for the first time, and a labor government removed explicit racism from immigration law in 1967.[175] National self-consciousness about these changes eventually precipitated a broad shift toward cultural independence. The trope of bodily authenticity certified the appropriateness of the new training for the cultural work at hand because of a wider concern to generate uniquely Australian arts. Thus, progressives increasingly identified with Aboriginals in their nationalism.[176] Aboriginals participated in this change by achieving greater visibility through protest that extended from achieving citizenship, and they had begun participating in the avant-garde arts, including dance.[177] The African American teacher and choreographer Carol Johnson founded a five-year training program, NAISDA (National Aboriginal Islands Skills Development

Association), for Indigenous students in 1975. Ultimately, this led to the establishment of the Bangarra Dance Theater in 1989, a renowned Aboriginal dance company.

The new position of Indigenous culture in Australia dovetailed with the idea that reproducing classical European aesthetics signified a perpetuation of colonialism. Thus, by seeking an authentic Australian dance as a way to gain significance within a transnational cultural circuit, organizations such as Dance Exchange configured colonialism as being a thing of the past. More recently, Scott Lauria Morgensen, writing on queer Indigenous studies, argues that "settler colonialism is naturalized when conquest or displacement of Native peoples is ignored or appears necessary or complete," a problem he identifies in queer settler communities.[178] From this perspective, Somatics practices can be seen to have participated, albeit unwittingly, in Australian settler colonialism. Yet, by interrogating this participation, we can see how the American expansionist underpinnings of the training transformed themselves in foreign contexts by presenting liberal democracy as a progressive development while affirming capitalist imperialism's inevitability.

Australia impacted the transnational network less visibly than the other hubs, yet for dancers there the relationships with the other centers affirmed Australia's position in the community. They connected most strongly with Manhattan, where the potential for innovation with Somatics seemed the greatest. Karczag performed Brown's choreography, Dumas connected with Tharp and Rudner, and Hassall first went to discover what she calls "the new dance," which she found attending a multitude of loft performances by artists such as Meredith Monk, Yvonne Rainer, and other Judson artists, including Trisha Brown and Lucinda Childs, while also studying at Julliard and performing in the Merce Cunningham Company.[179] For Dumas, New York remained a site of pilgrimage for young Australian dancers to encounter resources for innovation, while Karczag, leaving Brown's company, rejected New York's professionalization of Somatics, which she felt threatened the creative agency dancers had carved out in the 1970s.[180] As full-time faculty member in the Netherlands at the EDDC, she became a vocal proponent for Somatics as a source for innovation, publically criticizing the use of Somatics to recapitulate classical or modern aesthetics in line with a Dutch body in flux.[181] She taught workshops in all the transnational hubs I have mentioned, as well as many others. All the members of Dance Exchange taught as SNDO and thus benefited from the focus of Dutch Somatics on utilizing teachers from the transnational community. However, despite the rich discourse in *Writings on Dance* and the unique antipodean experience with the regimens in the 1970s, with the odd exception, Australia largely remained an outpost within the transnational network.[182]

Conclusion

The transnational network exhibited unevenness in the degree to which each geo-Somatics body signified beyond the local community in which it was cultivated. Interrelationships nonetheless catalyzed the symbolic meaning and the material conditions through which the regimens manifested in each hub. Through a dynamic set of connections, dancers sustained the underlying tropes that established the field and accessed necessary resources as late twentieth-century contemporary dance underwent local and transnational change. Crucially, dancers preserved the conceit of the natural body with its cumulatively distinct implementations of the rhetoric. By positioning itself as the center, New York's professional and innovative body resourced the network with varied pedagogies and choreographies, verifying the creative potency of connecting with natural corporeal capacity. New England's body in artistic respite, however, safeguarded against losing the connection with nature by providing a symbolic space beyond the reaches of commercialism and institutionalization. The socially critical British body failed to have the same reach as either of its American equivalents, yet emerging as it did through dispute with a conservative establishment, British Somatics epitomized nature's dissident potential for dancers from across the network. Similarly, by functioning as a vessel for discourses from foreign contexts, Holland's body in flux largely disappeared beyond the higher education in which it was cultivated. Yet the Dutch commitment to the transnational network provided employment for many artists and supported exchange between various contexts, enriching the overall discourse. While Australia's new frontier body largely affected only those artists that lived in or visited it, it nevertheless stood for the potential of Somatics to disseminate creative freedom to ever more unchartered geo-cultural territories.

The different symbolic and material functions of the geo-Somatics bodies changed in character and importance in relation to the phases of development articulated in chapter 1. In the 1970s, without substantial institutional backing, dancers verified the value of their marginalized efforts through the transnational scale of their venture. With its reputation of advancement, New York symbolized the potential of the regimens at a time when artists in various contexts were struggling to establish alternatives to modern dance. Meanwhile, British Somatics functioned as a conduit for resources from

New York through Dartington College, and X6 modeled the determination with which independent projects could be pursued in a hostile environment. In this same phase of early development, Australia justified the missionary zeal with which Somatics pursued its own expansionism. Then with commercialization and institutionalization, New England stepped in as a site to which artists could flee from the professional circuit to protect the value of Somatics. Similarly, through its separation from its own domestic dance culture, Dutch Somatics took up the role of an outpost for American innovation and a site of transnational exchange, when Britain closed its borders by asserting a nationalist contemporary dance culture in the 1980s. The emergence and shuffling of distinct roles within the transnational network maps the phases of development to which Somatics was subject. Yet the same topography constructed and retained the rhetoric of accessing universal individual creative freedom through the natural body.

We can see how well the transnational strategy worked for Somatics in the fact that great numbers of contemporary dance educators ultimately embraced the training. They invested in the idea that through the regimens, students accessed extracultural motile capacity as a practical foundation for unique unfettered artistic potential and unprecedented health and sustainability. By the twenty-first century, Somatics had spread beyond the West and found its way into a range of major dance training institutions. Programs now apply its analysis of the body to the very classical and modern training that Somatics was initially developed to resist, as well as drawing upon its approaches for novel movement invention.

Considering the diversity of ways in which Somatics emerged in various contexts, a reader unfamiliar with the training may find the belief that it is based on an essential universal body confusing. Yet dancers' ongoing investment in the rhetoric is not dissimilar to the pervasiveness of Western medicine. Many of us assume that the best treatment for a fracture, for example, is the same for all people wherever they are located because we are thought to share a basic skeletal structure with properties that have been discerned by science. Dancers worked on a similar principle when they configured Somatics as a means to rescue individual creative freedom from existing traditions, or as the optimum means by which to recalibrate existing vocabulary for new choreography. Yet to the degree that Somatics naturalized individuality, universality, and dissidence through the body, it compounded the ubiquity of liberalism in contemporary dance. Dancers therefore embodied postwar liberalism through the belief that they were developing critical projects from a blank slate, and this fomented an artistic culture that claimed to provide freedom from establishment constraints and provided the space to stage political and aesthetic critique. Liberalism not only sidestepped interrogation but also seemed to be the very basis from which critique was possible. By looking at concert dance in the next chapter, we will better understand how liberalism helped to smooth over the paradox between dancers' initial intention to critique institutions, and the eventual appropriation of Somatics by those same organs of power.

3

Somatics Bodies on the Concert Stage

Processing, Inventing, and Displaying

I opened chapter 1 with Leslie Kaminoff's quote from *Movement Research Performance Journal* that warned about the problems of faking "release technique." In the same issue, which focused on release as an approach to dance, Simone Forti protested that "there's so much life beyond letting go and flowing," indicating her distance from the current practices. Nonetheless, the term "release technique" emerged when contemporary dance, informed by Somatics, achieved success on large concert stages based on choreography that demonstrated the very qualities Forti described.[1] Large numbers of dancers subsequently pursued the skills associated with release-related regimens, and the training found its way into major dance education institutions. Establishments, which had initially repudiated Somatics, endorsed the aesthetics with employment opportunities and earning power. However, by the end of the century, as Forti's and Kaminoff's comments indicate, the institutionalization of Somatics prompted concern that outer appearance was displacing the focus on inner knowledge in training, and that broad choreographic possibility was being lost to a narrow set of canonized physical aptitudes and compositional approaches. In their opposition to these changes, some artists harkened back to the aims with which dancers had begun using the regimens forty years earlier. This chapter revisits the development of Somatics in the previous two chapters to examine its influence on and application to concert dance, focusing specifically on choreographic production in New York City. From its use as an exploratory approach valued in a small community, Somatics slowly became institutionalized through the aesthetics associated with the work of a few choreographers who became successful on a transnational scale.

Dancers in the 1960s had employed Somatics to establish creative agency by rejecting the choreographer's authority in new dance-making processes, and by the 1970s, dancers had corralled the idea of nature to synthesize creative processes, vocabulary, and modes of organization that they saw as comprehensively inclusive. Thus, in the United States the improvised work of

The Natural Body in Somatics Dance Training. Doran George, Oxford University Press (2020). © Oxford University Press.
DOI: 10.1093/oso/9780197538739.001.0001.

Steve Paxton, Barbara Dilley, and Nancy Topf built on the previous decade's experimentation in ways that were related to but distinct from Trisha Brown's and Forti's 1970s set choreography.[2] The next decade's artists drew attention to social identities that had been excluded by 1970s universalist claims. The 1980s East Village work by Ishmael Houston-Jones and Channel Z, as well as Yvonne Meier and Jennifer Monson, for example, asserted the value of individual difference. These artists also critiqued the institutionalization that was happening in this time period as Brown garnered success on large concert stages. In the 1990s, choreographic processes largely reinstated the choreographer's authority that Forti and her colleagues had initially rejected. Somatics provided the skills for dancers to fulfill the choreographer's vision, restoring company hierarchies.

With chapter 1 having already traced the historical development of the regimens and their core ideas, this chapter looks specifically at how choreographers worked with Somatics and how they interacted with dancers through the medium of Somatics-based physicality. Organized topically rather than in a strict chronology, I take up three distinct sets of choreographic strategies that were implemented in the making, presentation, and reception of dance. Avoiding any labels used extensively within the community, I propose "processing," "inventing," and "displaying" as analytical terms based on my perception of artists' understanding of their approach to choreography. These different strategies reveal not only changing conceptions of the dancer and choreographer roles but also the power relationships between them. By framing the strategies in relation to broader social changes, I trace the way that political liberalism was initially exercised through collectivism, then transformed into entrepreneurialism, and subsequently into a corporatized institutionalization of Somatics. In brief, I argue that beginning in the 1960s, dancers choreographed their experience of moving based on Somatics ideas in "processing," which seemed to provide a universal foundation for individual authenticity. Based on this approach, 1970s dancers cultivated anti-hierarchical collectivism in their concert culture. Through "inventing," they also produced what they felt were novel forms of dance based on knowledge afforded by Somatics experience. Even though these principles emerged in an overlapping milieu with processing, they powerfully embodied 1980s entrepreneurial culture and social change by providing methodology to invent individual signature vocabularies and stage new social identities. Finally, it was through "displaying" that choreographers ascended to 1990s institutional contexts with signature vocabularies based on the theatrical effects through which the other two strategies conveyed their ideologies.

Despite excursions beyond America to consider local differences and transnational influences, the primary focus on New York in this chapter capitalizes on the city's role as the symbolic center for contemporary choreography. I use Britain as a counterpoint to show how state funding, a distinct dance establishment, and other local conditions mediated the development of the work. To probe the nuances of institutionalization, this chapter also looks at a handful of alternatives to the dominant model of 1990s dance, tracing how other artists staged their own versions of Forti's objections. Examples include dances by Stephanie Skura, Stephen Petronio, and David Rousseve, as well as Eva Karczag's solo improvisation, and the intergenerational choral practice of British choreographer Rosemary Lee, whose work circumnavigated the impact of the transnational success of Somatics.

Processing: Choreographing Somatics Experience

Based on pedagogies developed in the 1960s, many 1970s artists established what they saw as a new definition in Western concert dance of the choreographer/dancer relationship by rejecting the distinction between the two roles. As the dancer and choreographer were collapsed into each other, one creative agent emerged whose identity was determined by the mode of training. Artists thus placed the performers' experience in the foreground, participating in broader subcultural trends that extended decision making to all those concerned. The milieu therefore saw its approach as cultivating antihierarchical collectivism in concerts that embodied the direct democracy seen in Somatics classes during the same decade. Because of these developments, Somatics enjoyed a mutually influencing relationship with concert dance for the rest of the century.

Somatics contributed to new choreographic ideas, and in turn, these ideas translated into procedures that influenced practice of the regimens. One of Steve Paxton's 1970s improvisations illustrates how his concerts dovetailed with and drew upon Somatics ideas. His position as a key critic of conventional choreographer/dancer relations also meant that he influenced many artists who staged their experience based on Somatics, so understanding his practice provides insight into the larger milieu. Paxton scheduled the dance in question to begin on his arrival at a New York venue directly after traveling from his Vermont home.[3] Removing a backpack and boots, he signaled the journey's end and the dance's beginning.[4] Taking a bus as a "warm-up" was one among several ways that he "investigated the mind of the dancer" by varying his preparation, a decision that also embodied the challenge to erase the separation between training and concert. By staging his choice of preparation as the dance's subject, Paxton replaced the choreographer's authority with the dancer's experience.[5] Furthermore, coming from Vermont signified nature's integrity in spaces beyond the city associated with the back-to-the-land movement. Paxton thus contested the artistic power structures associated with metropolitan culture by focusing on what he called "those who were seen to be the pawns in the game," and instead he charged the dancers to explore "the source and processing of choreographic movement."[6]

Forti similarly influenced the community by staging the consciousness of the moving body.[7] Her dances investigated what Banes calls "elements," including "balance, weight, momentum, energy, endurance, [and] articulation of the body."[8] Forti displaced what she saw as the outdated aesthetics of pointed feet and extended arms with task-like actions such as pulling oneself up an angled plane in *Slant Board*.[9] With a focus on the awareness of action, and the decisions about kinetic form being left to the moment of performance, Forti aimed to divest dance of anything "superfluous," following "questions of perception rather than questions of theater."[10] She choreographed the dancer's experience as one unconcerned with appearance. Drawing on her study with Halprin, in which the body was treated as "physical material" available for investigation, Forti's works, including *Slant Board*, reframed Halprin's pedagogy as performance.[11] Midcentury Somatics therefore contributed to the communitarian organization of concerts in the next decade, which seemed to foreground the individuality of dancers. This dovetailed with emerging Somatics pedagogy that insisted upon the intrinsic corporeal nature of kinetic skills, independent of aesthetics, and found solely through exploration.

By focusing on their experience of the moving body, Contact Improvisation (CI) dancers likewise staged the dancer's experience of moving as its subject. Novack argues that any concern with the outer form of CI was secondary to the tracking of changes in the body's relationship to gravity. By emphasizing kinesthetic awareness, she suggests that dancers reduced their risk of an unanticipated fall, which established processing as a necessary condition of performance.[12] She attributes an internal gaze, widely seen in 1970s CI dancing, to such demands.[13] In duets, the dancers connected their respective centers of gravity to each other from which they extended loose limbs to sense the floor and regulate the gradual spread of falling weight. The vocabulary therefore served the mandate to pay attention to gravity and momentum. Yet along with other behavior that represented the dancers' ordinariness, an internal focus also signified antitheatricality.[14] CI dancers insisted that they were performing "as themselves," concerned with the experience of moving rather than expressive or aesthetic protocols. Novack chronicles the rapid expansion of CI culture as a 1970s antihierarchical movement in which, like *Slant Board*, dancers staged direct democracy by performing the experiential investigation of physical principles.[15]

Nature represented a site at which control could be renounced for the dancer to discover new possibilities. CI and those trained in other Somatics pedagogies believed that they opened themselves up to new creative possibilities through their kinesthetic awareness of anatomy as it interfaced with terrestrial forces such as gravity. Novack suggests that CI, in particular, transgressed social norms through physical inversion and moving sideways while spiraling or curving, facilitated by a sensation of reducing control over the direction the body takes.[16] But she points out that the duet form redefined lack of control by insisting that "contact improvisation can teach an enjoyment of disorientation and a reconsideration of spatial associations."[17] CI blurred the lines between participation and performance, which affirmed for dancers the universality of the sense of self they felt they recovered from nature. The duet form therefore recycled the "natural universal individual."[18] With performances framed as the demonstration of an activity in which virtually anyone could participate, CI spread rapidly in the early 1970s, and the pedagogy was designed to avoid years of virtuoso training.[19] In the first ten years, Novack recounts inclusivity was valued, with the idea that any two people could dance together, which was underscored by the initial rawness of the form.[20]

The early transnational dissemination of Somatics also embraced inclusion of those coming from different kinds and amounts of training, even though the regimens fueled more conventional performer/audience relations. Strider and Dance Exchange, for example, fostered participation through education programs. Stephanie Jordan notes that Strider was the first British company to perform in nonproscenium settings and described their mission as wanting to "integrate the work of dance with everyday life . . . to make more contact than a mere performance can allow."[21] Similarly, Australia's Dance Exchange executed residencies outside of theaters to build audiences and plant the seeds for a dance community. By introducing nonprofessionals to dance that was ostensibly inclusive and universal, early British and Australian Somatics aimed to demystify concert dance. Anatomical Releasing, which strongly influenced both companies, provided a language and pedestrian kinetics that were accessible in a way that classical and modern dance vocabularies were not.[22]

The emphasis on participation in such performances extended to theories of viewership. Flux in the ideas about the meaning of performances helped to affirm the antihierarchical nature of the culture by replacing expertise with mutual enquiry. Reviewers wrestled with their role. For example, in responding to a performance of CI in 1977, Deborah Jowitt asked, "Can it be (ought it to be) defined and evaluated only in terms of how it feels to the participants, or can the opinion of an outsider (teacher, critic, spectator) be considered?"[23] She concluded that it is hard not to stratify the dances, confessing it is "impossible not to view as successful . . . transfers of weight and energy [that] are clear," but she insists that the ultimate value is in an empathetic response: "If the lifts are breathtaking it isn't because they look difficult or prepared, but because they look so easy, so in tune with my own pulse that, watching them, I am extended."[24] Reflecting on her potential bias, Jowitt signals the degree to which CI culture renounced the primacy of a spectator's experience, while validating her conviction that dimensions of self are elevated by the pleasure of viewing, further evidence of how CI was thought to enhance essential dimensions of the self. By blurring performance and participation, practitioners configured viewership as a vicarious kinesthetic experience. Novack reinforces this focus by insisting that "contact improvisation stimulates . . . the spectator to identify with the sensual, proprioceptive experience of the dancers."[25]

Along with CI, many other artists refocused attention on the dancer's experience in performance. Nancy Topf developed game structures performed by groups throughout the 1970s,[26] while Barbara Dilley, after leaving Cunningham's company, rather than teaching her own style, authored instructions for performance in order for dancers to "realize and clarify their own dancing selves."[27] Such work shared New York spaces, dancers, and reviewers with CI but, unlike the contact jam, depended on the cast having a level of sophistication in Somatics training, such that the concerts looked quite distinct from classes. In her 1978 review of Dilley's *Dancing Songs*, for example, Mona Sulzman admires the "delicately and subtly sustained group rhythm" that dancers such as Cynthia Hedstrom executed by virtue of a combination of Somatics, modern, and classical training.[28] Meanwhile, Topf worked with Daniel Lepkoff, Body-Mind Centering (BMC) teacher Beth Goren, Nina Martin, and Patti Giavenco to design games that cultivated the individuality of her dancers. She contrasted her spatially defined rules with the dimensions of the choreography over which the dancers had control, including "the dynamic and temporal aspects [which] are more open to the discretion of the dancers."[29]

Even though the rule-based choreographies required a level of skill from their performers that distinguished them from early CI, as procedures designed to highlight the Somatics emphasis on kinesthetic experience, they exhibited a number of principles in common with the duet form. The dances seemed to be antihierarchical because the performers made their own choices. The formality of the structures also claimed to connect the dancers with natural universal truths of form rather than marshal bodies within imposed culturally specific ideas. The dancers thus appeared to "find" themselves within the choreography, generating new social possibilities by taking risks.

British artists also staged processing, but their dances embodied the battle with establishment conservatism, with justification for the work framed by "New Dance" feminist discourse rather than the exploration of unknown potential. When Kirstie Simson improvised at X6 with skills learned from Paxton at Dartington, Emilyn Claid saw her as exceeding classical limitations on women, arguing that she has "no physical boundaries . . . no feminine pretense, no primness; she is out in the open, free from constraint."[30] Meanwhile, Chris Crickmay asserted the value of Miranda Tufnell's structured improvisation against disparaging press responses.[31] Tufnell worked with "a framework of suggestions,"[32] which, similar to Topf and Dilley, depended on training in Somatics and martial arts.[33] Battling press hostility, Crickmay recycled American CI ethics by positioning her work in opposition to "older forms," which also paralleled Claid's rejection of classicism. He insisted on the egalitarianism of Tufnell's work, which "rejects hierarchical or directive social relationships between one performer and another, and between performers and audience."[34] He wrote that she and her collaborator, Dennis Greenwood, are "no mere marionettes dancing to prescribed steps. They are thinking beings, constantly seen in the act of making choices."[35]

Notwithstanding transatlantic differences in their discourse, American and British artists similarly overlooked important aspects of their cultural specificity. Overwhelmingly white, they nonetheless upheld the universality of the possibility for dancers to access freedom by choreographing kinesthetic experience. This contradiction between the rhetoric and the dancers it served embodied an attitude identified by Banes as "essentialist positive primitivism."[36] She argued that Greenwich Village artists embraced African American aesthetics such as bent limbs, compartmentalized torsos, contrapuntal rhythm, emphasis on gravity, repetition, and improvisation, all of which signified "the concreteness of the body," as opposed to ethereal virtuoso Euro-American corporeality.[37] CI culture in the 1970s also initiated a comparison between its concerts and jazz music to insist on the value of improvising against set choreography. For example, reviewing a CI concert at New York's Kitchen, Stephanie Woodard argued that CI "is the closest thing that dance has to jazz."[38] By borrowing ideas from black culture, artists seemed to value what more mainstream dance ignored or denigrated, yet by framing the ideas as precultural, following terrestrial forces or "neutral" formal spatial and temporal rules, artists erased their use of African aesthetics, in a manner similar to the way that CI used martial arts.

By insisting upon the universality of their practice with the claim that they were accessing a precultural body, however, dancers working with Somatics in their choreography also exhibited a second idea about race underpinned by antiracist intentions. Banes argues that, unlike the radicals who valued racial difference, 1960s black and white liberals asserted equivalence by "deny[ing] racial and cultural difference in their fervor to gain equality for African Americans."[39] Artists who subsumed African aesthetics into universal ideas about the moving body therefore insisted that the ideas about black people against which racists railed were foundational truths for every moving body, which would have seemed to combat racism rather than erase cultural specificity. However, as Banes and Claid admit, neither 1960s Greenwich Village nor 1970s British New Dance addressed racial difference or the exclusion and marginalization of black dancers.[40]

Perhaps not surprisingly, then, referring to the Manhattan locale where many of the dances I have analyzed were staged, Dixon Gottschild argues that "'Downtown dance' . . . the loose, less structured, experimental form(s) that emerged from downtown Manhattan venues like Judson Church . . . is the code for white dance."[41] Woodard, by failing to mention the African American dance form that grew up alongside jazz music in her claim that CI most closely embodies the sonic tradition in movement, supports Dixon Gottschild's claim. Moreover, regardless of the sexualities of those who participated in 1970s CI and related dance practices, a comparison of the approaches with contemporaneous queer performance reveals the heterosexuality of the practices. For example, like CI, the San Francisco "Cockettes" cultivated an antihierarchical collective culture and sought freedom by opening themselves to disorientation in performance. Yet they did so by marking their often-naked bodies with exuberant signifiers of gender to contradict conventional heterosexuality.[42] By contrast, Somatics and CI depended on "performing modesty," evacuating emotional and sexual impulses to establish the scientific veracity of their practice. With the increased access to CI through the rapid establishing of its artistic network, participation of increasingly diverse dancers exposed the monocultural make-up of the community and its ethics.[43] Yet dancers understood their vocabulary to be based on "pedestrian" movement, despite the focus on disorientation and the need for specialist training for the choreography based on rule structures. The culture therefore seemed to espouse inclusivity, making it hard for dancers to critique the universalist claims put forward.

Nonetheless, developments associated with the 1980s challenged the universal claims of choreographing kinesthetic experience. East Village improvisation revealed some of the limits of inclusivity by highlighting a tension

between the cultivation of antihierarchical collectivism and performing individual and social identity. *Wrong Contact Dance*, staged in 1983 by African
Americans Ishmael Houston-Jones and Fred Holland, exemplified this critique by contravening what the dancers saw as tacit CI rules. Presented at
"Contact at 2nd and 10th," a large New York gathering of the CI community to
celebrate ten years of the form, Houston-Jones and Holland wrote a manifesto
to define how their dance failed to meet the conventions of the duet form:

1. We are Black.
2. We will wear our "street" clothes, as opposed to sweats.
3. We will wear heavy shoes, Fred, construction boots; Ishmael, Army.
4. We will talk to one another while dancing.
5. We will fuck with flow and intentionally interrupt ourselves.
6. We will use a recorded sound score—loud looping of sounds from Kung Fu
   movies by Mark Allen Larson.
7. We will stay out of physical contact much of the time.[44]

Houston-Jones and Holland embodied desire, fear, aggression, and resig-
nation by choreographing distance and proximity, opposition and collapse.
By grasping each other's clothes, pressing flesh against flesh, and sustaining
balances for long periods punctuated by sudden tussling, the dancers evoked
psychic intercourse more than the dispassionate observation of moving physical architecture. Appearing to follow erotic impulses by attempting to control
each other physically rather than following momentum, they insisted that attraction and repulsion are equally integral to investigating bodily motion as
gravity.

A comparison between *Wrong Contact Dance* and Paxton and Stark Smith's
duet on the same program reveals the African Americans' departure from
1970s ordinariness. As they had in the previous decade, Paxton and Stark
Smith averted erotic or emotional readings of their proximity by emphasizing the dance's mechanics. Barefoot and in a CI standard of loose sweats,
their mutually facilitated balancing and lifting followed a pendulum-like motion that conveyed natural momentum; stillness was a tipping point rather
than a pregnant pause, and the dancers' internal gaze displayed that they
were sensing moving weight or the structure of a balance. Dancing ten years
after the birth of CI, the pioneers did reflect a specific aesthetic, yet it was by
extending a style Novack calls "the dancer is just a person."[45] This trope distanced 1970s aesthetics from epic modern dance narratives by insisting on an
objective relationship to the scientific reality of ordinary human kinetics. It
was with quotidian amusement, like a knowing smile, that Paxton and Stark

Smith commented on inadvertent associations brought forth by their dance. Yet along with the audience, who shared their amusement, they did so by recapitulating modest ordinariness, by considering such connotations from a distance.[46]

While Houston-Jones and Holland's intervention related to broader CI trends, they also participated in an East Village critique of minimalist aesthetics that, building on 1970s experimentation, were now finding a place on large concert stages.[47] The improvisation ensemble Channel Z, for example, who all trained and danced in CI contexts, experimented with integrating actions of social affront but performed as if they were neutral movement.[48] Company member Paul Langland recalls: "There was a lot of release work and being nice in the 1970s . . . with white yoga pants, etc. By 1980 I became interested in expanding the range of pedestrian actions to include . . . slapping, screaming, groping each other. . . . But quotes were placed around these actions so they could be seen in their pure form."[49] Along with Martin, Randy Warshaw, Diane Madden, Petronio, and Lepkoff, Langland expanded CI's unpredictability by initiating, amplifying, embracing, and transforming the meaning of socially coded action. In duet, ensemble, and solo, the company staged familiar scenes of social interaction, such as arguing with or greeting someone, but not as pantomime. Instead, they focused intently on the movement, thereby allowing viewers to see such actions in a new way.[50] As in *Wrong Contact Dance*, social reference added psychic momentum to the movement of weight, contesting and expanding the existing assumptions about how to dance, and insisting that dancers can investigate more than the awareness of gravity and momentum.

The increased expertise in performance techniques on which Houston-Jones and Channel Z depended prevented the broad participation of untrained dancers. Novack argues that a similar shift took place in the CI network when dancers developed virtuoso skills and no longer wanted to duet with beginners, and concerts and training also became increasingly distinct.[51] The dexterity and uniqueness of the dancing and the aesthetic reflexivity they staged exhibited a shift in priorities that demanded commitment to a professional milieu. Bill T. Jones, who incorporated CI into his work, defended his career aspirations, insisting that to survive as an artist he had to "suit the ladies out in Iowa and also the young intellectuals in downtown New York who write about you and help you get your reputation."[52] Yet, East Village artists exhibited hostility toward such moves because the press tended to focus on a single artist's creative genius when they covered a dance concert, and dancers such as Houston-Jones, Stephanie Skura, and Yvonne Meier felt they functioned as collaborators.[53] Anticommercial ethics therefore emerged, not to claim that dance should be free from financial concerns, as was the argument among some CI dancers,[54] but to protect what they saw as creative integrity against the pressure to achieve critical repute and communicate to large audiences.[55]

With inclusivity threatened by professionalism, dancers sought to affirm their creative independence from commercial ethics by reasserting in their work the centrality of the dancer's experience. Channel Z did this by choreographing a space for failure, which recalled the process-based orientation of investigating movement protected from the concerns of presentation. While dancing for Cunningham, Neil Greenberg recalls being confused by a Channel Z concert in which dancers tried moves that they seemed to botch, despite the fact that some of them were also dancing for Brown.[56] Although unable to comprehend it at the time, he later learned that investigation was integral to the work. As a trope, failure verified compositional unpredictability, promising surprise, while insisting that the work was not marketable, thereby reformulating the 1970s rejection of theatrical concerns.

The difference between these works and the 1980s work of British company DV8, also indebted to CI, reveals how artists like Houston-Jones and Channel Z deployed the dancers' experiences as a foil to commercial ethics. In DV8's homoerotic duet *My Sex Our Dance*, Lloyd Newson and Nigel Charnock choreographed an ambiguous view of gay male sexuality that critic Anna Kisselgoff saw as a bleak vision in which "homosexual tendencies cannot exist without accompanying brutality."[57] Like Houston-Jones, DV8 represented urgency by foregrounding how the performance was taxing for the dancers. As Kisselgoff observed, "They really do wrestle, get red in the face, pant and groan from the effort and strain."[58] Yet the imperative of theatrical display, instituted through 1980s British state support, began to strongly influence DV8's social commentary.[59] DV8 provided seamless athleticism based on CI skills and themes that built on 1970s New Dance politics.[60] Their engagement at the Brooklyn Academy of Music, about which Kisselgoff wrote two years after the company formed, attests to the speed with which they began international touring and the professionalization of their productions. Meanwhile, in a context that disparaged accessibility and display, dancers in the East Village affirmed that they had not refined their performance for commercial viability. They made it explicit that they were engaged in decision making while performing and thereby processed their ongoing experience of moving, which was visible in the smaller venues where their dances played.[61]

In its opposition toward commercialism, the East Village spawned many contexts in which artists could perform experimentation. The weekly Hothouse improvisers exchanged their practices with fellow artists through informal presentation. Yvonne Meier and Jennifer Monson used such contexts specifically to further commentaries on social context by emphasizing interpersonal emotional entanglement. They choreographed cultural impropriety as if it arose from natural impulses that coursed through the body. For example, in a 1988 Hothouse showing, Monson and Meier began with arrhythmic torso undulations, throwing their heads into vomiting motion, followed by awkward taxing activity, like repeated manic springing with outstretched arms while bent forward. Their dancing appeared to be the inevitable result of bodily impulses that flouted rather than capitalized on social reference.[62] They constructed a body of natural unwieldiness that could break through conservative social mores.

Through continued recourse to the natural body, Meier and Monson participated in a discourse that, similar to CI practitioners a decade earlier, erased the specific character of the culture against which the intervention was being made. Novack asserts that by embracing physical loss of control, CI dancers in the 1970s had contravened a specifically white middle-class sense of propriety embedded in what she calls "American theater dance."[63] African American social dances had long incorporated inversion, for example, in the lindy hop, suggesting that it signified differently for those practitioners. By performing disorientation to "reconsider spatial associations," CI dancers embraced cultural otherness to disrupt a white tradition.[64] However, to the degree that inversion got naturalized through CI rhetoric about bodily mechanics, the influence of Africanist aesthetics was erased, along with the whiteness of the culture being critiqued.[65] Similarly, by naturalizing the body-psyche through which 1970s aesthetics were rejected, Meier and her colleagues risked concealing the white middle-class value system they were critiquing, and universalizing their cultural position. The changes to the staging of the dancer's experience in the 1980s reveal how liberal discourse shaped the possibilities of contemporary dance in a way that marshaled artists to frame their projects in universal terms through Somatics rhetoric. Acknowledging cultural specificity therefore often seemed oppositional to the project.

Despite these problems in their discourse, however, East Village and CI dancers made some important gains through the idea of universality and their focus on process. By maintaining the primacy of the dancer's experience, they embraced various axes of identity that were previously marginalized in dance.[66] CI dancers reconceived bodily capacity, including disabled dancers who had previously had little access to concert dance. Ann Cooper Albright insists that because of the focus on process, which she calls "the how rather than the what," disabled dancers did not have to fulfill a prescribed ability.[67] Alito Alessi, who developed accessible CI pedagogy, insisted on the naturalness and normalness of Emery Blackwell's movement, a dancer with cerebral palsy. Despite the difference in Blackwell's lexicon from those without his diagnosis, Alessi affirmed the disabled dancer's embodiment of CI using the rhetoric of nature. Alessi asserted that exploration must not be confined to an established vocabulary, yet such inclusivity broadened the notion of a universal body, compounding liberalism's natural basis and progressive potential.

Alongside the reinvention of bodily experience to resist commercialism, dancers also reasserted kinesthetic processes as a choreographic tool against the traditional hierarchical structures of companies using Somatics. From the 1980s onward, veterans such as Forti, Paxton, Simson, Karczag, Julyen Hamilton, and Laurie Booth established themselves as virtuoso solo improvisers who benefited from nostalgia for experimentation focused on process, a nostalgia fueled by the new efforts to codify Somatics-informed vocabulary. By staging their bodies and artistry as irrevocable, they modeled innovation independent from conventional career trajectories, seeming to sustain antihierarchical collectivism by insisting that commerce or a single choreographer must not displace the primacy of the dancer's experience. By avoiding forming companies based on their movement style, soloists benefited from low overheads. Yet they capitalized on an entrepreneurial arts culture in which their reputations were marketable.[68]

In virtuoso practice, the failure that affirmed the primacy of the dancer's experience in Channel Z's work transformed into a mastery of unpredictability. Artists staged their unique bodily knowledge through improvised performances. Paxton, for example, insisted that by hearing with his body and moving distinctly in each concert, "change, adaptation, or interpretation," which scoring and recording had robbed, were restored to his performances of J. S. Bach's *Goldberg Variations*.[69] Meanwhile, Claid endowed Simson's improvising with a value not available to dancers in traditional companies, describing her as a "powerful physical presence that could never be contained within the constraints of contemporary dance."[70] Simson, like Paxton, contrasted the staging of the dancer's experience with procedures that depend on a known or set artistic product.

Karczag established the exceptional artistic potential of improvisation with her responsive, open, supple body, one that was revered in her community and admired by critics for three decades.[71] Karczag performed advanced bodily knowledge through the unflinching concurrence with which she embraced incongruous changes as she folded, oscillated, swept, jerked, flinched, collapsed, lurched, extended, and hesitated. Fluctuation in her focus of attention resulted in rapid multidirectional shifts similar to Houston-Jones's reworking of CI.

The complexity and speed of change appeared to be more than someone could register consciously. Jowitt likened her dance to dreaming, describing the way myriad images flicker across Karczag's motion with the ambiguity of sleep's dramatic landscape. Like Meier and Monson, and unlike Houston-Jones, who decisively ruptured modest performance, Karczag's gestures seemed fueled by unbidden bodily impulses. Reviewers saw her riding a frontier of sensory experience, because, although her gaze was not internal, it remained within her kinesphere.[72] Seemingly unperturbed by incompatible demands of her motile journey, Karczag presented herself as a virtuoso of the experience of the moving.

Also asserting the value of investigation, some choreographers reformulated processing within ensemble dancing. For example, with convictions similar to Simson's about the shortfalls of contemporary dance, the British choreographer Gaby Agis resisted the establishment imperative that shaped DV8's work.[73] In works like *Touch Un-site,* she emphasized her dancers' experience of moving.[74] Insisting that her casts' training in Skinner's work "allows

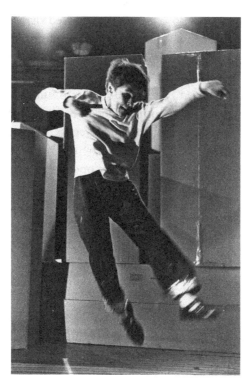

Figure 3.1. Yvonne Meier in *The Shining* in 1993.
Photograph by Donna Ann McAdams.

them to have an immediate response, an immediacy . . . [that] enhances the . . . awareness and ability to respond to space," Agis directed dancers to move slowly with eyes closed.[75] They performed in various nontheater spaces, representing the strong responsivity of their bodies to the architecture that they occupied. Shifting from large activity to small detail, similarly to Karczag, Agis choreographed changes in awareness in a series of activities to exemplify "the dancers' embodied experience of these spaces."[76] Restful contemplation followed frenetic action, a contrast heightened by the dancers' proximity to the audience.

Developing audience proximity further, Meier choreographed direct contact with her dancers in her early 1990s work *The Shining*.[77] Extending the interpersonal impropriety developed in Authentic Movement to her audience, Meier staged excessive intimacy and disturbing disregard.[78] She and her company of East Village colleagues guided small audiences through a dark maze, where they were physically manipulated into dancing and even violated in frisking dances or left bewildered, watching other audience members get embroiled in exceptional behavior.[79] Meier thus reasserted the ideas in processing by procuring audience participation in the experience of moving.

Meanwhile, British artist Rosemary Lee composed visions of inclusive community with intergenerational casts of dancers and nondancers. Her mixed casts performed mutual care to embody and represent an embracing sociality. Based on the participation of untrained dancers ranging from toddlers to seniors, critics characterized Lee as creating community well-being.[80] Many of the choral works relied on a motif of dancers listening with their ear placed on each other's bodies, building on attentiveness developed in rehearsals. Using the kind of reflective exercises seen in Anatomical Releasing, her dancers cultivated what they understood as openness toward themselves and each other. The action, which resembles the hands-on practices of Somatics, conveys a sensibility of contemplative mutual care. Figuratively and literally, the cast listened to the "nature" of each other, creating a sense of belonging through collective acceptance. Like Meier, Lee reimagined participation as a theatrical effect, violating the protocols that, as we will see, came increasingly to dominate 1990s Somatics vocabulary.

Inventing: Somatics Sources of Novel Movement

Dances that exhibit principles I have grouped under the label "inventing" initially aimed to manifest the same antihierarchical collectivism of CI and other related process-oriented choreography. Yet, although staged in overlapping milieux, the performances maintained a distinction between choreographer and dancer roles and strove to establish a unique signature in both vocabulary and compositional approach. To resolve the inevitable tension between the choreographer's authority and the centrality of the dancer's experience to collective ethics, artists worked to stage nonhierarchical relationships. Rather than collapsing the dancer and choreographer into one identity, as with processing, inventing redefined the dancer as a collaborator with an explicit decision-making role. The work emphasized the intellect of dancers applying their skills at processing physical information to compositional structures arranged by choreographers. The strategy therefore embodied the ideal of direct democracy and displaced what were seen as the hierarchical structures of modern and classical dance companies.

The focus on new vocabulary and composition resulted in choreography that achieved levels of complexity that clearly demanded specialist skills. Nonetheless, by drawing on a pedestrian vocabulary and style, the dances initially exhibited the broader 1970s claim that Somatics accesses bodily movement common to all humanity. The choreography theorized a universal anatomical origin for its motility, replacing participation with a kind of conceptual or vicarious accessibility often achieved through simple gestures or task-oriented movement. Within the structures that choreographers authored, dancers created complexity from ordinariness, thereby staging their intelligence, while also occupying a collaborative role. In this sense, by virtue of the apparently ordinary source of the vocabulary, choreographers reframed themselves as facilitators, and dancers asserted their creative intelligence. Through inventing, artists therefore extended liberalism by affording individual creative freedom to the dancer.

Trisha Brown's 1972 *Primary Accumulation* illustrates both the central role of Somatics to inventing and the difference between inventing and processing. In a grainy black-and-white film of the dance shot from above, Brown lies horizontally, filling center frame, lifting her right forearm so that it's perpendicular to her elbow, with her hand remaining flat as it was on the floor.[81] She could be minimizing muscular tension while sensing the elbow joint like Somatics students, and indeed Elaine Summers's Kinetic Awareness work informed the vocabulary, visible in the apparent effortlessness with which Brown adds simple actions in this and other dances with an accumulating structure. Writing about the work, Banes insisted, "the beauty of the dances rests in the choice of gesture . . . simple, compatible and articulate . . . and also in their execution which has little to do with virtuosic dance and everything to do with presence . . . tenderness, and honesty to the raw gestures themselves . . . seeing ideas em-bodied."[82] The gestures fold into each other, overshadowing the transparency of 1,1+2,1+2+3, etc., revealing a complexity beyond the layperson, despite the component actions appearing not to be based on specialist training. As in Paxton's improvisation following his bus trip to the performance, Brown initially performed her dance, and therefore arguably fused the choreographer and dancer roles. However, rather than staging her dancing self as producing vocabulary by investigating an idea in performance, Brown executed a premeditated structure with largely predictable kinetic outcomes.

Through authorship, 1970s Somatics-informed choreography contributed to the decade's changing gender mores, and as the century progressed, artists returned to inventing as means to renegotiate other axes of social identity. Along with Brown, Simone Forti and Rosemary Butcher used Somatics to contest entrenched gender roles by asserting intellectual authority over movement, rather than emotional authority as Graham had seemed to do, and they also validated the dancer's intellect. These moves reflected how women were proclaiming their intelligence and taking up leadership in the Equal Rights Amendment movement aiming to outlaw sex discrimination. Similarly, the three artists choreographed gender equivalence by contesting the idea that men are more intelligent and leadership-oriented, while also disputing the reliance of choreographic authorship upon power differences. Furthermore, like the staging of the dancer's experience, they also staged bodies as knowledgeable rather than as objects of desire by making visible a concentrated, perfunctory execution. Performed in "art galleries, lofts, other churches, and various other non-proscenium spaces,"[83] Brown and others intentionally turned their backs on the trappings of concert houses, aiming to avoid "conventions that are hanging all over the theater space: preconceptions that aren't present outdoors or in a gallery."[84] Likewise, distancing herself from the stage, Forti saw some of her work as minimalist sculpture, which was similar to Butcher, who thought of her dances as the temporal and spatial embodiments of geometrical form in a visual art idiom.[85]

In her 1970s "mathematical pieces," including *Primary Accumulation*, Brown accumulated and reordered what appeared to be components of pedestrian kinetics into complex dances, the ordinariness of which Brown verified by insisting, "I can't . . . fake extravagant movement."[86] She linked pedestrian vocabulary and Somatics, maintaining that in *Primary Accumulation*, for example, "movement . . . has to be natural, comfortable, and simple."[87] Modern dance's polarized representations of male and female found themselves replaced by a neutral body that Brown constructed using low muscle tone, passive weight, and sequencing based on flow. Jowitt observed, "Everything [Brown] does seems to . . . flow out of her without any tension. . . . [T]he adjustments in her body are fluent, natural looking . . . using just as much time, space, and energy as she needs and no more."[88] Halprin's Alexander-like open-ended approach underpinned Brown's ease in *Primary Accumulation,* which she developed by "using it . . . like a warm-up exercise, accumulating to as far as I had gone the last time, in a . . . relaxed manner with no goal."[89] Yet, while her casual manner affirmed the naturalness of her neutrality, the precise but poetic accretion of gestures asserted her authorship. Brown's dancer from the late 1970s, Lisa Kraus, called the choreography "natural movement not extending beyond a normal range of motion, in which body parts were lined up creating right angles peppered with rhythmic detail."[90] The fact that the movements seemed ordinary highlighted the structures that Brown invented to sequence them, thereby emphasizing the predetermined plans that were then executed.

In her solos, Forti also expanded ordinariness by contending that it is underpinned by ontogenetic, terrestrial, and phylogenetic realities evident in infant, pedestrian, and animal kinetics. The identity she constructed appeared as equivalent to, but an intelligent guide for, the audience through what Banes calls the "defamiliarization" of everyday action.[91] Banes traces Forti's dances from the early 1960s, when she was "finding dance . . . in the common-place . . . dissecting ordinary movement,"[92] until the mid-1970s, when she built upon "crawling, animal movement, and circling [walking],"[93] seeming to recover efficiency in kinetic detail and performing the complexity of simple action. In the 1974 dance *Crawling,* Forti offset deceleration and seamless con-tinuity with accentuated weight shifts. Banes observed "analytical intelligence at work as Forti examines each term in the sequence."[94] Forti also staged an-imal motility as a common evolutionary inheritance, integral to biped skeletal structure. Deducing how human bones best emulate the structural kinetics of lizards, bears, frogs, and other species, she cultivated seamless transitions from one species to another, asserting the intrinsic nature of the patterns to humans with ideas like Todd's.[95] Gradually altering her placement, she shifted between species, using weight and momentum to construct natural motile logic and aesthetics. As in Brown's structures determining the sequencing of movements, Forti's compositions did not explore a process in performance, but instead showed how the body could transform within a predefined order of images.

Butcher saw herself as facilitating her dancers' intelligent connection with nature by shaping, with spatial and temporal accenting, movement they produced. Like Topf, she gave her company "formal" prompts, maintaining "what I have to offer [is] a task form. . . . they [the dancers] must . . . move in their own way."[96] So despite setting her dances, Butcher insisted they emerged collaboratively. As Crickmay puts it, "The choreographer sets up the conditions within which the dance can be 'found.'"[97] Butcher believed that aesthetics arose from anatomical function, replacing classical and modern lexicons with walking or running.[98] *Pause and Loss* (1976) combined settling together, leaning on each other, and departing with similar but never in-unison timing. Repeated hopping with a low front-extended leg highlighted the flocking and dispersal as the numbers of those doing the action increased and dwindled. By 1980 in *Spaces 4*, a lean or embrace interrupted walking, running, sitting, and lying, with occasional soft lunges or spirals into and out of the floor. Through her compositional simplicity, Butcher persuaded her audience that her vocabulary arose from, rather than being imposed on, her dancers.[99] Through her careful temporal and spatial arrangement, she made her input visible.

Butcher and Brown rechoreographed their approaches for concert houses beginning in the late 1970s, resulting in substantial changes in the appearance of their work. In contrast with Forti's solo approach, they adapted their vocabulary for the different demands of the proscenium arch. Butcher's touring works, such as *Traces* (1982) and *Flying Lines* (1985), maintained an understated nonathletic gender-equivalent vocabulary. They enthralled audiences with temporal drama by amplifying acceleration and stillness. Brown's *Glacial Decoy* (1979) intensified rhythmic irregularity with incongruous small gestures that initiated weight or direction changes and shimmying shoulders or elbows appearing from skips or jumps in which the torso rode calmly on the legs. Linda Small describes the languidness as "stream-of-consciousness movement, in all its astonishing nonviolence," calling the dance "an elegant, casual form" with "disjointed movement dialogue."[100] The dancers diverged, collided, and regrouped as shared vocabulary surfaced from unrelated movement and direction. Yet alongside the unpredictability, similar to her 1970s manipulation of ensemble presentations of *Locus* and *Sololos*, Brown asserted artistic authority by underlining her choices with moments of unison.

Although Brown reinstated an artistic hierarchy by devising vocabulary and sequencing, the dancers affirmed their jurisdiction over the new vocabulary by developing individual strategies for its execution. Reviewers celebrated such individuality; Small contrasted Kraus with "Brown's postmodern clones who cannot match her fleshiness,"[101] while Jowitt delighted in "the pleasure of watching two women in unison as much as their differing temperaments permit: Karczag constantly silky and resilient, Brown given to small eruptions."[102] The orientation of the dancers in space further connoted the dancers' ownership of the vocabulary. Directed toward 360 degrees rather than a frontal view, spectator pleasure seemed incidental to the movement, embodying the disavowal of a concern with appearance in Somatics. At the same time, the pedestrian origins of Brown's vocabulary progressively disappeared. The likelihood of audiences imagining themselves in the movement, like they might have done with the accumulations, diminished. As we have seen, reviewers now described the dances' appearance rather than the movement process. Furthermore, their focus on Brown's signature vocabulary and the valuing of dancers' unique execution made evident the lessening interest in antihierarchical collectivism in line with a broader cultural turn toward an ideology of individual achievement through merit-based success.

East Village artists responded to similar social and artistic changes, also building on 1970s vocabulary. Yet by privileging experimentation over careerism and sustaining collective ethics, they embodied the individualistic culture, but in a way different from Brown.[103] Dancers reveled in irreverence toward a theatrical status quo, staging provocation that reflected changes in feminist strategy. As the culture wars dawned, these artists asserted the power of spectacular sexual difference, flaunting the female body as a desiring subject rather than a sexual object. Cindy Lauper's successful version of the song "Girls Just Wanna Have Fun" released in 1983 captured the new aesthetics, which took pleasure in the dazzle of the spotlight by reworking 1970s insights and flouting old ideals of beauty with staunch individual feminine difference.[104] East Village dancers similarly embraced spectacle, reformatting Somatics to forge what they felt was unique vocabulary that dramatized the ways in which marginal bodies were being framed. They thereby expanded the inclusivity of their dances, particularly through the inclusion of new visions of the feminine. Committed to experimentation and opacity of meaning, in events such as Hothouse, the close-knit community interrogated the possibilities for social commentary by delving into what they saw as the vicissitudes of the body.

With a loss of optimism reflected in the broader culture by the defeat of the Equal Rights Amendment, expressions of frustration and anger became an appropriate response. Continuing work already begun in the late 1970s, Pooh Kaye staged urgent repetition of Forti's lexicon. Kaye's all-female company jumped obsessively on all fours; slammed into walls, the floor, and each other; and displayed bodily endurance, which, in ways different from Kaye's predecessors, rejected traditional femininity while also relying on Somatics. By using skills from Anatomical Releasing and Skinner classes, such as sequencing through joints and low muscle tone, Kaye and her dancers, including Meier and Monson, minimized injury with a logic not dissimilar to Forti's use of velocity in the polar bear–like swinging of the head.[105] With speed and repetition, Kaye staged a vigor similar to that seen in Houston-Jones and Holland's surging force, as well as Meier and Monson's explosiveness. Choreographing desire, frustration, aggression, and convulsion, artists threw a powerful spotlight on individuality.

In spite of sharing similar kinetic tendencies, artists asserted the idea of individuality in unique approaches that they invented using the differences in the regimens on which they drew. Houston-Jones's interpersonal consternation contrasted with Meier's intrapersonal emphasis. Like Brown had done in her mathematical pieces, they both authored instructions, yet differences arose between Houston-Jones's and Meier's methods through the training on which their dances relied. Houston-Jones and Holland constructed individuality relationally, contravening CI by replacing harmoniousness with confrontation. In *Them,* Houston-Jones instructed his dancers to embody "tentative, fragile attraction . . . like the two sides of a magnet . . . drawing you together . . . pushing you apart" in what he called the "circle duets."[106] By contrast, the prompts for Meier's kinetic perplexity pushed against personal aesthetic and psychological limits. She and Monson aimed to marshal corporeal impulses through Meier's *No No Scores*, which broke the precepts of Rainer's "No Manifesto" and, like Houston-Jones, rejected 1970s aesthetics.[107] She constructed and confronted a familiar self in dances of fear and pain, or pure

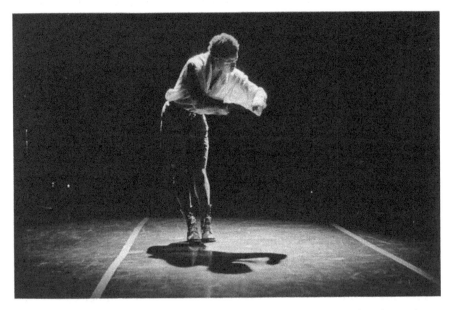

Figure 3.2. Ishmael Houston Jones in *The End of Everything*, performed at The Kitchen in 1988.

Photograph by Dona Ann McAdams.

aggression, and she sought inspiration in the obscene, hysterical, ugly, bizarre, and sleazy, among others. Houston-Jones and Meier both asserted their authorship by emphasizing individuality and claiming to launch their dancers beyond constraint into unrepeatable frenzied vocabulary propelled by the unconscious.

Although Meier initially felt CI and Somatics faithfully fulfilled inclusivity, she subsequently staged her own intervention into the new practices.[108] She rejected Skinner's language of physical integration with her *No No Scores* by replacing natural imagery and nurturing adjectives, such as melting or floating, with words like exploding that she then coupled with body parts. She distorted CI's logic of natural flow by choreographing conflicting states in different body parts like "running, interrupted by rhythmical frenzy" or "fierce rhythm possesses the spine." Meanwhile, Houston-Jones asserted individuality by contesting both conservative and leftists agendas.[109] *New York Native* writer Robert Sandla castigated the contradictory ideas in *Them* as a homophobic staging of "sex and violence, love and death, as irredeemably intertwined."[110] He bemoaned the new uses of CI resulting in a "slam, bang, smash, heap, tussle, and grapple" where "support and concern [are] purposefully lacking."[111] Houston-Jones refused to comply with leftist imperatives to represent positive images of marginalized subjects, but he also drew attention to the foreclosure of possibility in mainstream gay culture as much as CI by reflecting on the demonizing of queer bodies by conservatives. Despite continuing to stage the dancers' experience of moving, both artists asserted their authorship as inventors through their glaringly idiosyncratic approaches. So even while they sustained collective ethics in their experimental milieu, authorship based on distinct individualism underpinned the artistic critiques.

In their defiant attitudes toward large theater, East Village dancers often relied on audience familiarity with the vocabulary shown on those stages that they then critiqued in their use of failure and provocation. Viewers understood that Channel Z dancers were contravening modest performance with interpersonal affront, pop culture, and dance history references, while the space for failure affirmed their experimental aims. The company members therefore distanced themselves from the refinement seen in Somatics-informed work for large stages. Falling, scuffling, and colliding replaced CI seamlessness, while erupting, tripping, and flailing worked similarly in relation to Brown's effervescent precision. Many dancers also looked directly at viewers, compared with the internally focused, downcast eyes of 1970s dancers and most Somatics work seen on large stages. In *Wrong Contact Dance* the duo conveyed confrontation with their gazes, as did Houston-Jones in his masturbation solo in *Them*. Channel Z dancers frequently embodied characters, or

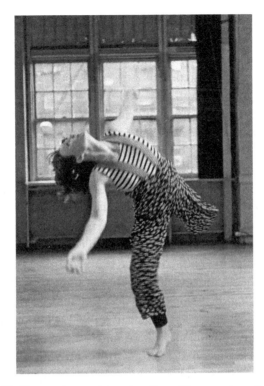

Figure 3.3. Jennifer Monson improvising at an Open Movement session at PS 122 in the 1980s.
Photograph by Dona Ann McAdams.

they shifted from inner sensing to an outward focus and back, thereby challenging the sense of the dancers as a continuous persona. Monson and Meier also alternated their gazes in a way that signified their sourcing impulses but also showed their awareness of others. Change in the use of the eyes positioned dancers as social subjects rather than physical masses in the throes of falling or ascending with gravity. Like the codes of failure and social reference, the legibility of this tactic relied on familiarity with the internal gaze of the previous generation and the intimacy of small theaters.

Monson embodied her politics as physical experience rather than textual themes by frequently improvising on a daily basis with artists such as Meier, DD Dorvillier, and John Jasperse. Together they investigated kinesthesia rather than psychology or social message, asking, "What physical sensations can we arouse in relation to each other?"[112] Like Houston-Jones, Monson rejected any limits on identities such as woman or lesbian, for which she became notable during the culture wars. She examined instead the vulnerability raised by the devastation of the AIDS crisis, the risks entailed in protesting against the attacks on reproductive rights, and the fight for lesbian visibility through the groups ACT-UP and the Lesbian Avengers. Synthesizing 1970s androcentric and gynocentric gender equivalence, she "wanted to be as powerful as a man but there was a rawness and a vulnerability that I really valued."[113] Her comment suggests that raw vulnerability complicates male strength, an idea she pursued with the kind of androgynous vocabulary seen in her duet with Jasperse in *Finn's Shed* (1992). Of the dance Cooper Albright observes, "strong, explosive movement, does not preclude a softer, more tender dancing."[114] Professional soccer tackling served as one of the motifs for developing the vocabulary, which recalls Paxton's use of apparently nonaesthetic Aikido skills combined with the increased vigor of 1980s CI.[115] Jasperse and Monson ran and threw themselves at each other, crashing safely into the floor. Based on different relationship dynamics, Monson infused a similar vocabulary with sexual energy for a 1993 duet, *RMW*, with Dorvillier, which I will return to later in the chapter.[116] In choreographing social commentary by intertwining Somatics and personal relationships, Monson was not alone, and the approach was largely supported in her milieu.[117] In all these stagings of social relationships, the choreographers made it evident that they were following shared sets of rules that had been invented and agreed upon rather than simply processing an image or physical state. In this way they participated in the same reimagining of Somatics that was taking place on the mainstream stages in Brown's work. However, their embrace of more aberrant, wacky, and marginal character types sustained the political radicality of earlier Somatics investigations.

Meanwhile, in Britain, inventing tended to embody liberal dissidence mediated through the political ideal of accessibility.[118] This happened a decade before American CI turned to "diverse communities," probably because New Dance sought to reach people seen as marginalized.[119] A concern about conservatism and exclusivity influenced British artists who sublimated rather than emphasized discriminatory practices in dance. For example, Lee aimed to overcome contemporary dance elitism, while Candoco codirector Adam Benjamin argued that disability provides an invaluable critique of narrow aesthetic ideals.[120] Both choreographed idealized inclusive communities in which the dancers were interdependent and collaborative, rather than provocative individuals. They influenced and were influenced by British "community dance," which promulgated inclusive ethics and emerged from the drive toward participation underpinned by educational and therapeutic aims.[121] In the late 1970s, state arts funding also focused on education and by the 1980s envisioned the direct involvement of audiences as a key to a healthy arts culture.[122]

Lee developed her aim of putting diversity on the concert stage while teaching community classes in the rapidly expanding early 1980s community dance programs.[123] By disbanding the bodily ideals in professional training, she wished to represent each dancer as equally valued.[124] Early 1980s New York experience also influenced her approach, which reflects how British artists brought ideas home from visits to America. She invented vocabulary that avoided stratifying dancers as more or less competent because of their age, training, or physical capacity.[125] Lee sourced 1970s CI practices by ceasing to use counts and developing kinetic forms based on sensory exercises that do not rely on precise repetition. With movement that focused her cast toward how each dancer feels, similar to CI, she challenged established aesthetics, defining her vocabulary against skills that demand years of classical or modern training. As Lee puts it, she rejected concerns like "how high they could lift their leg."[126]

Similarly, Benjamin cultivated responsiveness using weight and breath, with which he insisted dancers achieve authenticity in contrast with exclusive classical vocabulary.[127] Disabled and nondisabled dancers used Somatics in inventing movement that demanded skill from all the participants, theorizing disabled dancers as intelligent bodies that contributed to vocabulary that did not fit into existing techniques designed for the nondisabled.[128] Dance critic Chris De Marignay refers to Candoco's "extraordinary choreographic solutions," which used CI ideas of "leaning, falling, and supporting."[129] With leverage, gravity, and momentum, disabled and nondisabled bodies forged interdependent identities. Candoco therefore choreographed a kind of integration in which they both challenged the idea that competent dancing depends on the exclusion of disabled dancers and resisted the prevailing representation of disabled people as incapable.[130]

In Britain, the integration through inventing of bodies that had largely been excluded from dance depended on a 1980s dance boom.[131] Following the paucity of opportunities for independent projects in the 1970s, the boom was characterized by a rapid growth in funding and programming on which artists capitalized by working with Somatics. Under pressure to create innovative, accessible, and participatory projects, Somatics came to fuel dancers' creative labor for initiatives that would attract funding, programming, and critical acclaim. Like DV8, Candoco met the aesthetic protocols of the concert house circuit with virtuoso vocabulary, while Lee depended on the regional dissemination of contemporary dance, instituted by a statewide national agenda.[132] Like the East Village artists, Candoco and Lee utilized the strategy of inventing to put forth progressive and inclusive political values.

America saw a comparable dance boom during this period in which the creative autonomy through which dancers initially asserted their agency became a requirement for employment in "pickup companies," a term used by mid-1980s New York dancers for what Randy Martin describes as "a group of dancers assembled for a single run of performances."[133] While these pickup companies featured dancers' individuality and utilized compositional approaches in which dancers devised and contributed much of the movement material, they presented works that were clearly conceived and rehearsed by a single choreographer. This would eventually lead some dancers to question the politics of the collaborations for which they had contributed their creative efforts. These kinds of shifts portended the erosion of collaborative dance making as dancers found themselves displaying an empty idea of agency through vocabulary in a way that reinstated the choreographer's superiority.

Displaying: The Theatrical Effects of Somatics

A third way that Somatics entered onto the concert stage, one that I call "displaying," largely resulted from choreographic strategies that artists developed to negotiate institutions. This new approach, however, conflicted with processing and also with the initial aims of inventing. As artists began to reengage with theatricality, following the intense critique against it mounted in 1970s Somatics aesthetics, they found that it was not necessary to foreground the dancer's experience of moving or sustain collaborative equality to exploit the creative potential of the regimens. Therefore, despite having first asserted the ability of choreography to resist concert dance's focus on appearance, artists informed by Somatics began to focus on visual meaning, increasingly verifying their worth as authors of the dance through the appearance of the moving body. Consequently, choreographers gained even more access to large concert houses and established their approaches within powerful training institutions through composition and vocabulary that were singularly attributed to their creative labor, relegating the dancer's explicit role to an interpretive rather than more collaborative one.

In Skura's 1987 dance *Cranky Destroyers,* for example, we begin to see how, by exploiting the visual effects of Somatics, artists moved into more mainstream theatrical contexts. Initially, using Skinner-influenced exploration, Skura linked her interest in the idea that the unconscious is inflected with an intrinsic bodily logic informed by dream images, creating ambiguous symbolic content.[134] To expand creative flow in coaching the dancers, she theorized physical impulses as a source for free association, like Karczag. Recalling Meier's *No No Scores*, she sought contradictions between movements by asking them to interrupt internal censors. She also included scenes from her and her dancers' dreams, paralleling Channel Z's use of theatricality, and contributing to a collaborative company culture.[135] East Village colleagues danced in her work, using aptitudes from CI and Somatics to "give in" to rather than direct their dance.[136] Through consultation with her dancers, Skura amplified what she saw as their unique qualities, from which she chose and adapted vocabulary to emphasize individuality in the final composition.[137] Furthermore, *Cranky Destroyers* exhibited the vigorousness, obsessive repetition, and sudden change in direction that characterized the East Village critique of the aesthetics on large stages. Yet Skura insisted that such vocabulary fulfilled the theatrical conventions against which it was initially developed. In the *British Dancing Times*, Jack Anderson describes with delight "six dancers [who] waggled their heads, hobbled laboriously . . . and collapsed to the floor. There were quivers and shivers, creepings . . . sprintings,

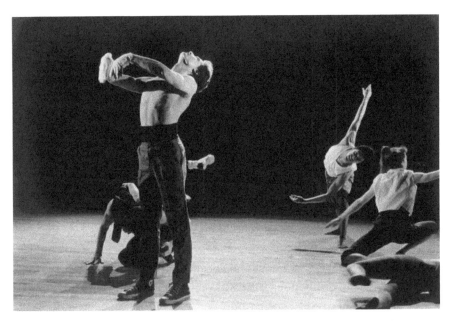

Figure 3.4. *Cranky Destroyers* choreographed by Stephanie Skura, in collaboration with the dancers, at its premiere performance at PS 122 in 1987. Performers in photo (from left to right): Benoît Lachambre, Stephanie Skura, Brian Moran, David Roussève, Margery Segal, and Debra Wanner.
Photograph by Dona Ann McAdams.

and flingings about."[138] He theorized the vocabulary as surprising, compelling, and innovative for a transnational context.

The demands of large houses, however, forced Skura to reassess theatricality as utilized within displays of East Village irreverence. To achieve the kind of visibility demanded by large theaters, she forfeited evidence of either the dancer's experience of moving or the dancer's intelligent contribution to the choreography, thereby setting new parameters for the dance's reception. Thus, New York critic Elizabeth Zimmer suggested that "courageously . . . she's in open waters," in reference to the premier of *Cranky Destroyers*.[139] Skura wanted to avoid the kind of confusion Greenberg experienced when witnessing Channel Z's embrace of failure, so she modulated what dancers learned, for example, instructing them to cut every third movement from a busy section or asking them to involve the arms or execute a lift that nearly occurred. In these ways *Cranky Destroyers* replaced failure with quirky virtuosity. Combining classical lines with impossible tasks, they displayed a comic kind of expertise.[140] When they turned, balanced, or leapt, the dancers pushed into the floor, extending the limbs distally to create shape rather than sense their "interiority." Zimmer describes them as "virtuosic on their own terms, athletic, highly mobile in their upper bodies, and [yet] rarely constrained by conventional behavior."[141]

As part of the emphasis on how the movement looked, Skura's dancers learned movement that she selected from videoed improvisations that they had done. Then, after piecing sections together, Skura edited further.[142] Like Karczag, Monson, and Meier, Skura resisted the symmetry and linearity of classicism, yet she also satirized formality with a clearly premeditated if unpredictable structure.[143] Upstage duets counterbalanced downstage solos, which were related in kinetics and timing. Dancers even walked to a place on the stage to be lit by a spot and began to move. Along with uncanny spatiality, the vocabulary seemed to deride while embodying a presentational dance idiom: dancers thrust their pelvises, twitched their legs, and bounced their heads or arms, directly facing the audience. Cincinnati's Marty Munson comments on how the vocabulary in *Cranky Destroyers* offered something new and distinctive from the strategies we have seen in processing and inventing when he observed that "as faithful as she is to the integrity of each dancer . . . Skura's works have an overall style. . . . Movement seems to emphasize a similar quirkiness and interest in gesture. What begins as one movement frequently ends as another, adding the feeling of surprise and unpredictability."[144] By framing the vocabulary as signifying, rather than embodying, individual innovation, reviewers confirmed that the emphasis on displaying removed the agency that dancers had achieved by staging their own experience of moving and asserting their creative input within the chore-ographic process. Zimmer further reveals what was seen as important when, talking of Skura's offbeat composition, she assured her readers: "you won't get bored."[145]

Once it had been transformed into appearance value, however, critics reframed provocative individualism as a generalized and liberal cultural dissidence, thereby losing the East Village critique of cultural homogeneity. Anderson seemed to appreciate her rejection of minimalism, asserting that al-though Skura's choreography "could be described as an abstract dance . . . such a bland description would fail to convey . . . its extraordinary eccentricity."[146] Yet he read kinetic anomaly in *Cranky Destroyers* as asserting undifferentiated creative freedom and also as an attack on the conventional proprieties associ-ated with a musical work such as Beethoven's Fifth Symphony to which much of the dance was set.[147] Anderson reports he had to "think about esthetic de-corum," concluding, "why should we allow convention to dictate what sort of choreography is or is not appropriate to certain types of music," talking of the "musical irreverence with cleverly designed choreographic messiness."[148] When the work toured, regional American critics built on and referenced Anderson's ideas.[149] Now codified for large theaters, the East Village break with propriety signified universal nonconformity in which "the personalities of the performers are allowed to shine through."

Cranky Destroyers universalized individual provocation, embodying a problem to which artists who pursued success within the conventional dance touring circuits were bound: the imperative to fulfill theatrical conventions often undermined their critique.[150] Skura had depended on her dancers' input for the unconventional spacing and movement, sourced from their responses to internal impulses cultivated with her prompts for improvisation. But to make idiosyncrasy legible beyond the East Village, she transformed the strategies of processing and inventing into a form of display. So as artists re-engaged theatrical protocols, the impact of Somatics changed even though the same rhetoric endured. The new choreography still staged new dancer identities compared with classical and modern choreography; however, as *Cranky Destroyers* reveals, it reflected a new identity for the choreographer of the work.

Whereas Skura's provocative individuals invited the gaze, reveling in trans-gression, Brown's dancers displayed a resolute lack of concern about being looked at while taking pleasure in the experience of moving, building on the choreographer's earlier rejection of concert stages. Through compositional strategies and kinetic effects that were recognizable independently of par-ticular dancers, Brown constructed a nonchalant dancer. So although, like

Skura, she never codified vocabulary as a technique, Brown nevertheless created a set of kinetic forms and codes to represent nonchalance regardless of who was dancing.

The nonchalant dancer also superseded the limitations of spectacular femininity by displaying intellectual prowess in her play with gravity and skeletal structure. Sharp, rapid changes in direction, often barely altering location, shocked the dancers out of the direction in which they were falling, which blistered feminine ethereality with intellectual acuity through the deft performance of unpredictability. Although focused on weight and momentum, the dancers kept resurfacing with poise and attention so as to relocate for the next action rather than allowing themselves to "go with the flow," as Novack suggests had been typical of CI in the 1970s.[151] Percussive breaks in the hips took the dancers forward, backward, or sideways, reorienting them to tasklike continuous motion and resisting a romantic resolution of gravity invited by the lilting quality. In *Glacial Decoy*, the soundtrack of dancers' footfalls contributed to an obsessive quality along with nonsensical patterns created by rebounding flexion in the elbows and knees, but soft execution in the detailed design and jolting rhythm suggested contemplation rather than mania. The women seemed to repudiate while contemplating feminine display by effortlessly performing a mentally demanding lexicon in proscenium arch trappings and glowing white fabric. Yet, unlike the collaborative thinking dancer of the 1970s, Brown's new vocabulary demanded technical masters of the form, which she stretched between sensuousness and spatial authority with her signature vocabulary.

Brown asserted analytical prowess and virtuoso unpredictability at a distance from the classical idiom, establishing the nonchalant dancer by *displaying* a lack of concern with *display* using Somatics aptitudes. Ballet dancers achieve elevation and extension by pushing down into the floor with their feet while externally rotating the legs and lifting the upper body while stabilizing the pelvis. Friction with the floor prior to a leg gesture creates energetic release and length in the limb, translating into climactic lightness and elevation. This gives dance a heroic quality along with turnout and a torso position that Melanie Bales says conveys "high emotional effect." She contrasts such efforts with the markedly relaxed body employed by "Judson dancers."[152] Continuing the Judson focus on a relaxed body and working with anatomical logic, Brown found the "natural, well-coordinated instinctive ability to move" that she sought as opposed to the affected quality of a "puffed out ribcage" in classical and modern dancers who, she insisted, could not "do a natural kind of movement, not even a simple one."[153] The making of *Glacial Decoy* coincided with company changes as Brown began working with dancers such as

Kraus who were trained in Somatics as well as modern and classical regimens. Yet the company focused on internal anatomy, emphasizing function as they directed their bodies, seeming not to care about display.

Brown's ability to take forward several compositional strategies from *Glacial Decoy* helped to establish her signature. She demonstrated nonchalance as a set of kinetic effects that were also applicable to men and through which heterosexuality could be sublimated without evacuating sexual difference. By referencing ordinariness and privileging no stage area, Brown disengaged from the spatial, temporal, and energetic stratification through which compositional poignancy normally provides the differentiating drama between the sexes. The men's occasional display of physical strength when lifting women appeared mundane in *Set and Reset*, which treated every action with indifference.[154] Ramsay Burt argues that the dancers' apparent disregard for the audience and the horizontal dispersal of sublimated masculinity into an overall structure resisted the construction of dancing men as bravura. He insists that in the original staging, Petronio and Randy Warshaw's "powerful contributions are redistributed into the texture of the piece as a whole, through the way the dancers' gaze is contained, and through an overall, decentralized structure."[155] Dancers fall and catch themselves or each other while limbs rarely extend fully except to navigate tipping weight or elongating a swing. Legs hang with weight as dancers lift their knees with ease, dropping feet into gravity that pulls the leg and pelvis, reverberating in the torso, and shifting them in a new direction with uneventful skips. The composition amplifies such motile insouciance with pathways that seem incidentally related such that Burt insists "the piece avoids . . . development or climax through . . . uniformity of incident and . . . continuous, fast, strong but free pace." He describes this as the "antithesis of the balanced, symmetrical grouping found in, for example, the ballets of Petipa."[156] Yet slipping impossibly in and out of unison, the dancers displayed the coordinated nature of the choreography's mercurial unpredictability. Interchanges between dancers, such as when one dancer would fall and be caught at the last moment by another, even while one or both dancers were looking away, also asserted compositional control. With moments that frame casualness as intentional, Brown insisted that the sublimation of sexual difference within nonchalance is something that the dancers achieved by displaying her choreographic strategy.

Despite the seeming indifference to display, Brown laced her ordinariness with sexuality, supported by the way Somatics projected sexual nature onto black bodies and movement traditions, while erasing such investments. Recalling her 1970s sensuousness, reviewer Marcia Pally argues, "*Set and Reset* has the beginnings of an erotic edge."[157] Brown's subtle use of the erotic recalls the broader shift in the 1980s when artists asserted the integral nature of sexuality to the body. However, in contrast with Houston-Jones, for example, and to avoid gender asymmetry and theatrical provocation, Brown dispersed the erotic throughout her vocabulary and composition. Nevertheless, despite staging androgynous sensuality in what she saw as her "one phrase fits all genders" approach, she still naturalized masculinity.[158] Brown avoided what she saw as "undignified" movement for the male body and modern dance "clichéd images of . . . muscular male movement."[159] By placing hypermasculinity at one end of a spectrum, Brown indicates she aimed to avoid men performing overly feminine dance at the other end, which confirms Burt's suggestion that *Set and Reset* integrated Warshaw and Petronio's "power."

By contrast, in his company, Petronio amped up the association between sexual perversion and dancing men by reveling in undignified movement and staging queer masculinity. Along with artists such as Michael Clark, Javier De Frutos, Russell Maliphant, and Mark Morris, Petronio updated classical and modern vocabularies largely rejected by his predecessors.[160] He synthesized these with Somatics in what Claid describes as lyrical male homosexuality.[161] British dynamics influenced Petronio through his connection with Clark, who, Burt argues, "follow[ed] in the tradition of gay artists . . . [that] intentionally debase . . . high art"[162] and incited a conservative establishment by infusing ballet with transgressive symbols as part of culture responding to "a climate of AIDS activism."[163] Using flexion and inward rotation in his own debasement of balletic line, Petronio, who performed for Clark, similarly indulged in referencing and contravening classical propriety, rejecting Brown's heterosexual ordinariness.[164] By incorporating classicism as a feminine sign of queer male sexuality, Petronio capitalized on the way male heterosexuality is brought into question on the dancing stage.[165] He represented queer masculinity through men's embodiment of spectacular femininity, which theorized a dancing identity that had been excluded by minimalism's rejection of spectacle.[166] In so doing, Petronio portended work by Neil Greenberg, John Jasperse, and Tere O'Connor, all of whom choreographed male femininity with Somatics as a sign of queerness.[167]

Like Brown, Petronio displayed his choreography using a recognizable vocabulary. With contained viscosity in *Full Half Wrong* (1992), rather than ripple, the dancers sequenced through their joints to full extension and snaked along the torso from the pelvis to the head. Petronio's vocabulary embodied Susan Klein's objection to "letting go," which reflects his investment in her technique. He also absorbed various idioms, creating incongruity that Jowitt describes as "slippery grace," which connects with Klein's claim that her approach is applicable to all styles.[168] Petronio dancers displayed erotic feeling through dynamism, causing Kisselgoff to marvel not at the performers "baring either breasts or bottoms," but that they "always appear to be living on the edge. Whiplash is the word to describe the propulsive power on display,"[169] a sentiment with which Nicole Collins agreed, describing Petronio's work as "aggressive, stylish, athletic, and highly sexed."[170]

In a further recapitulation of Brown's concert stage work, Petronio presumed the unilateral applicability of his vocabulary for both sexes, a strategy that brought its own problems. For example, the female soloist opening *Full Half Wrong* introduces dancing debauchery with gestures reminiscent of Nijinsky: her head throws back and with bedroom eyes her foot slaps and rubs the ground. She could be a boy being a girl as she writhes, holding under her thighs, waiting for penetration and then arching as if satiated, teasing the audience with her disembodiment of conventional femininity through queerly male seduction. Yet with their transgression of masculinity in the male body, men upstaged her homosexualization of the male gaze, so even if the women escape old-fashioned feminine sexual availability as symbolic queers, they do so only as a chorus for the men. In this way Petronio's mixed company reinstated gender asymmetry by universalizing the gay male body as the origin of artistic critique through sexual provocation.

Despite the distinct achievements and limitations in the dancing identities they constructed, by having their dancers display their ideas, Brown and Petronio both reinstated the power relations that were initially displaced with Somatics in the 1970s. With little control over the meaning they performed, the dancers faced a problem that Cooper Albright insists women face more generally because they "are always on display and yet often they are never really in control of the terms of that representation."[171] Although Brown constructed an identity that was unconcerned with the demand for spectacle by asking her dancers to emulate the appearance of indifference, she replaced collaboration and the intelligent dancer. Her company went from fulfilling instructions in the accumulations *Locus* and *Sololos* to learning set material.[172] Furthermore, Senter insists that in the 1990s the appearance of the repertory, achieved by learning roles from video, replaced ideas with which the dances were created;[173] the company valued the look achieved with Somatics rather than other forms of dancer intelligence.[174] Similarly, Petronio's gay male dancers seemed to take control by homosexualizing the male gaze, yet their provocation depended on mastering vocabulary. So despite the skill the dancers demonstrated, the identity they represented overshadowed their experience of and agency in exploring the dancing. Brown's and Petronio's displaying idealized their dancers rather than staging learning, discovering, and potentially failing, so the dancer's agency was largely banished from the stage and returned back to the studio training from where it had initially been unleashed.

As Somatics became more a set of skills that served as a resource for executing vocabulary rather than being integral to the identity staged, dancers drew on training techniques such as ballet initially rejected by the milieu in which Brown and Petronio had developed their work.[175] From the 1990s onward, Brown and Petronio's companies conceived of the dancer's role in this way, and some dancers trained classically alongside those using Somatics.[176] This marked change in the training approaches on which the company drew, accompanied by their focus on mastering the vocabulary, reinstated the choreographer's authority.[177] Dance critics followed suit, representing Brown and Petronio as the creative font of the work, no longer remarking on the dancers' individuality. Jennifer Dunning represented Brown as a singular artistic genius, "indisputably one of the most influential choreographers to come out of . . . Judson Dance Theater . . . having developed a style that has clearly left its mark on many younger choreographers and dancers."[178] Consequently, Banes's earlier insistence that Brown discovered rather than invented dance was forgotten. When writers represented Brown as a collaborator, it was now because of her work with famous artists working on her sets, accompaniment, and lighting rather than the dancers.[179]

In the early 1990s, Petronio, like Brown, was already represented as the single creative origin of his style, despite using Somatics-trained dancers,[180] who contributed to the artistic process in a similar manner to the development of Set and Reset. Petronio taught phrases that his dancers developed.[181] Company member Jeremy Nelson recalls, "He would show us something once and we had to make our own version of what we had seen, or we would make partner work based on a specific premise."[182] Yet Collins enshrined Petronio's choreographic superiority in her reviews of Full Half Wrong, insisting, "The distinctiveness of Petronio's choreography owes a great deal to his own idiosyncratic movement style," even verifying his company's quality by remarking on the dancers' ability to embody Petronio's way of moving. She suggests that the "prodigiously talented performer[s] . . . plunge headlong into [Petronio's] vernacular with the abandon of native speakers."[183]

To the degree that vocabulary informed by Somatics became recognizable through its codification, the idea of cultural specificity in kinetic forms pushed against the conceit of individuality dominant in 1980s inventing. At the same time, it erased or misrepresented influences from other traditions through the Somatics idea that inherent bodily capacity underpins individual innovation. Yet as Brown's work became broadly recognizable, some African

American choreographers began to assert the association of softness and flow with white contemporary dance. For example, due to his use of Somatics aptitudes, David Roussève's African American colleagues characterized his 1997 *Whispers of Angels* as "white dance,"[184] even though it can be clearly linked with black American modern dance.[185] Roussève's dancers exhibited kinetics evident in Brown's work such as emphasizing and following weight, and in Petronio's such as combining full extension with 360-degree dimensionality and using different levels. Yet they performed Ailey-like sumptuousness, such as reaching into space with a high releasing sternum, conveying a black spiritualist quality distinct from Roussève's white contemporaries. Ailey's characteristic tension and athleticism gave way, however, to languid ease, which 1990s company dancer Julie Tolentino recalls was achieved with Klein Technique.[186] A focus on anatomy produced seamless motion, circulating sensuality through the body, dispersing dramatic punctuation in the phrasing by avoiding sharp beginnings and endings. Nevertheless, Tolentino's experience of the milieu in which they worked adds credence to the charge that Somatics signified whiteness. She and the rest of the company, who had trained at the Ailey school, joked about their background with the awareness that jazz aesthetics were at odds with the conventions of contemporary dance. They accessed a lexicon associated with black culture by subsuming its presentational appearance with Somatics. In this way they expanded on both Ailey's and Houston-Jones's achievements by claiming new territory for African American dance traditions within a white-dominated context.

Although Roussève and his dancers used Somatics in ways that were meaningful for them and the large community of practitioners and viewers who followed their work, the transnational success of Somatics precipitated various forms of institutionalization, which resulted in Somatics often being imposed against artists' own sense of authentic expression. The experience of Phoenix Dance, Britain's first black contemporary company, exemplifies this problem.[187] Eager to nurture black dance in the wake of racial unrest, the British state encouraged a practice based on the idea that New York is the artistic center. The white American artistic director of Phoenix, brought in against the dancers' wishes as an Arts Council of England funding requirement, employed Roussève to work with the company alongside his colleagues Bebe Miller and Blondell Cummings, who were commissioned to choreograph repertory based on their work with Somatics. Yet while the African American artists fulfilled an establishment vision of black contemporary dance, their aesthetics conflicted with the local Northern English Jamaican immigrant heritage upon which Phoenix dancers drew. Christy Adair argues that the work resulted in "confusion for the dancers, as their success had been

based on their . . . performance of work that . . . drew on their cultural specificity."[188] Rousseve also recalls discomfort among company members about
his approach.[189] Thus, to attract state support, companies found themselves
displaying idealized identities of difference by fulfilling a broad agenda of participation mediated by the establishment imperative of technical excellence.
Reigning over these various forms of success was the identity of the choreographer as the origin of the work and its guiding artistic genius.

Conclusion: Nature, Artistic Rigor, and Economics

This chapter has traced how distinct aims, resulting from the social and artistic forces with which artists engaged, contributed to an aesthetic diversity
in Somatics-informed choreography. Multiple values and commitments, revealed through the analytical lenses of processing, inventing, and displaying,
shaped concert dance culture across the development of Somatics practice
from the 1970s into the 2000s. These included the contexts in which choreography was presented, how the vocabulary was produced and understood, and
the definition of the dancer and choreographer and the relationship between
them. On the one hand, individual artists such as Karczag exhibited principles in opposition to dominant norms of technical excellence and conventional company hierarchies. She staged her experience of moving as a creative
agent, one that combined dancer and choreographer roles. Her decisive use of
vocabulary evidenced her artistic dedication, as did her decision to work on
the fringes of contemporary dance, capitalizing on the greater intimacy with
audiences that small venues afforded. With a generous use of parallel, inward
rotation of the hips; collapsing in the elbows, knees, and spine; and hyperex-
tension in all those same joints, she distanced herself from classical feminine
display, demonstrating rigorous specificity and a sophisticated understanding
of concert dance language. Her approach, however, sometimes disappeared
in the discourse on nature, as when Jowitt described Karczag's suppleness as
being like an "infant."[190] She represented the artist as divesting her body of
culture rather than making a cultural intervention, which erased her incisive
wrangling with aesthetics.

Analyzing concert practices through processing, inventing, and displaying,
I have therefore tried to recuperate the cultural labor that artists invested.
Furthermore, this chapter identified how different approaches interfaced with
economies of presentation and dissemination. Most of the 1980s East Village
work I considered insisted on the experimental value of staging the dancers'
experience of moving. East Village artists also emphasized the collaborative

development of new vocabulary, which I called "inventing." Because they refused to fulfill a model of dance that was legible to booking agents, however, their work rarely moved beyond their local milieu.[191] Yet by modulating East Village ideas for their visual effect, which I defined as "displaying," Skura achieved broader dissemination than her colleagues such as Meier, Monson, Houston-Jones, or Channel Z. Nevertheless, because she depended on a collaborative relationship with her dancers and did not codify a vocabulary, Skura never enjoyed Petronio's level of success, an artist who paraded his love affair with spectacle by incorporating classicism. Brown, however, gained even greater acclaim with a vocabulary that became idiomatic of Somatics. By the 1990s, both she and Petronio had virtually branded their vocabularies, which were canonized as transnational contemporary dance ideals. Meanwhile, exploiting their claim to novelty in a different manner, Candoco developed a methodology that, by demonstrating innovation and technical proficiency, fulfilled British establishment contemporary dance ideals. Exhibiting the central principles of inventing, the integrated company offered unique skills to establishment-endorsed artists who were commissioned to choreograph new repertory for them. In a different approach, against the new demands of dance establishments, solo improvisers like Karczag, Paxton, and Simson rarely booked large venues but secured a transnational reputation by reinventing ideas associated with processing.

Value, associated with the size of audiences that choreographers reached or the aura of artistic rigor that work accrued, filled the contexts in which Somatics-informed dance circulated with tension. Brown's softness, and the flow she shared with Petronio, became associated with greater funding, programming, and critical support than Houston-Jones's skirmishes or Meier's explosions. Some East Village artists felt that support eluded their work because it was not "safe" enough for booking agents, which fueled the self-perception of the milieu as a space that nurtured integrity.[192] Meanwhile, Karczag rejected large concert stages because she felt that the focus on spectacle undermined the dancer's creative agency. She shared this sentiment with Paxton[193] and left Brown's company in the early 1980s, opting to foreground what she saw as her artistic integrity as a dancer.[194]

Yet to the degree that the discourse on nature concealed the cultural labor in which artists were engaged, the focus on artistic integrity overshadowed the impact of commerce on the organization of dance concerts. For example, Karczag forfeited the support that came with large spaces to avoid the construction of her moving body as an object of spectacle. Yet Wendy Perron, another Brown dancer from the 1970s,[195] infantilized Karczag's dependence on intimacy. Perron commented that, although she marveled at the concentrated labor visible in Karczag's detailed dancing, she wanted her to make "more grown up choices."[196] By linking an ability to communicate to large audiences with artistic maturity, Perron masked the economics that shaped dance viewership in a discourse on sophistication. Meanwhile, East Village artists felt they would have to dumb down their work to access large theaters, and solo improvisers like Karczag and Paxton saw a potential in proximity that was foreclosed by the proscenium's visual economy. So for some choreographers, artistic integrity seemed to depend on disavowing success. The discourses of nature and rigor obscured how these different strategies not only emerged under distinct economic, social, historical, and geographic circumstances but also shared in the ideals of liberalism by defining creative freedom against the encroachment of commerce. As my analysis of these examples makes evident, it is possible to arrive at a different solution than artists have tended to proffer as a way to recover the aesthetic diversity. Rather than expand the concept of nature or pursue artistic rigor, we need to pay attention to the myriad ways in which the Somatics idea of nature has been modulated to tackle different circumstances.

Conclusion

Understanding the Focus on Authenticity

This study has traced the relationship between training, dissemination, and choreography within a small community that identified itself as concerned with experimentation in contemporary dance. Applying insights about the body gleaned from earlier in the twentieth century, this group of artists and teachers slowly consolidated around their mutual disapprobation of modern and classical training regimens and their eager interest in exploring new paradigms based in the body's anatomical truths. Referring to this aggregate of overlapping practices as Somatics, I have argued that dancers worked to achieve an unencumbered individuality that contrasted markedly with the more authoritative imposition of aesthetics in classical and modern concert dance. By focusing on the experience of dancing, Somatics encouraged practitioners to connect with their "unique" embodiment of natural principles and to retrieve an authentic self that was thought to be integral to the physical body. This notion that the dancer embodies individual authenticity by accessing a natural body is probably the major contribution that Somatics has made to Western concert dance compared with, for example, the technical excellence in the idealized vocabulary of classical ballet or the codification of emotional expression in modern dance. Yet, despite the seemingly progressive thrust of Somatics, dancers, in their pursuit of individual authenticity, actually fulfilled postwar liberal ideals that were central to American expansionism and that permeate contemporary capitalism. The postwar American government justified military, economic, and cultural expansion by insisting they were protecting and propagating a universal right to individual freedom; dancers invested in the same idea by touting, as universally applicable, the notion that individual creative freedom can be accessed through functional imperatives of the body. This study consequently argues that Somatic authenticity embodies a late twentieth-century capitalist ideal of propagating universal individual freedom.

In chapter 1 I chronicled how dancers revolutionized training with the belief that they were connecting to universal bodily truths in individually unique

The Natural Body in Somatics Dance Training. Doran George, Oxford University Press (2020). © Oxford University Press.
DOI: 10.1093/oso/9780197538739.001.0001.

ways. With the theory that any dancer can achieve an authentic sense of self, Somatics developed through three phases. Initially established as a collective antihierarchical culture beginning in the 1960s, dancers reworked Somatics toward entrepreneurialism in the 1980s, and by the end of the twentieth century, the practices began to embody corporate culture, and institutions had appropriated the ideas cultivated independently in the two prior phases. Yet despite these changes in the training, practitioners continued to believe that they were achieving an authentic sense of self by connecting with essential bodily truths. Chapter 2, by tracing the transnational dissemination of Somatics training, connects the theory of universal individuality to American expansionism. With its focus on an authentic sense of self, Somatics engendered the liberal ideology that became important after World War II when America became a superpower. Yet, while the spread of Somatics depended on a flow of culture outward from New York, dancers in other contexts seemed to access intrinsic creative freedom via natural properties of the body. Wherever the regimens took root, dancers implemented them in unique ways that fed back into a transnational discourse, seeming to affirm both the universal relevance of the training and the training's ability to cultivate authentic self-expression. Chapter 3 analyzes how, using Somatics-trained bodies and related ideas, artists represented liberation from oppressive aesthetics and cultures on the concert stage. Through shifts in the conception of the dancer's identity, they choreographed a changing conception of the dancer that paralleled the development of neoliberal capitalism. By staging universal individuality in a diversity of ways, artists affirmed their creative freedom. Yet the dances embodied economic and political changes that were reflected in the continual reinvention of Somatics as it transitioned from antihierarchical collectivism to an entrepreneurial pursuit, and ultimately to an embodiment of corporate culture through its widespread institutionalization.

My analysis poses a problem for artists who have committed their lives to developing the training and for the large community of dancers now using Somatics. If the central contribution of the approach to contemporary dance is a sense of authentic individual creativity and natural physical autonomy and yet this embodies liberal capitalist ideals, artists seem to be robbed, theoretically at least, of the independence from commerce and access to artistic critique that Somatics promises. As a result, some artists are negotiating the appropriation of their practices and considering how they might continue to resist institutional hegemonies through Somatics. Although an analysis of their various approaches is beyond the scope of this study, I intend to validate the value of the labor of those who cultivated Somatics and to suggest certain possible ways of moving beyond this current dilemma.

If we wish to push against the imposition of ideology and aesthetics in the way that artists initially intended in their use of Somatics, we must track the cultural values being instituted now that the approach has been institutionalized. My account of the changes in training suggests that dancers' sense of agency depended not on accessing an essential physical nature, but on contesting the material and cultural conditions through which they were subjugated. The institutional success of Somatics clearly evidences this assertion. For example, in the 1990s, when artists were struggling to meet funding requirements in a corporate arts culture, choreographers depended on the ability of their dancers to invent vocabulary, yet the dancers were not accorded the value accrued to choreographers through the credentials of making a dance. Even in the earlier phases of development, when Somatics enjoyed greater independence from institutions, the racial and other marginalizing projections, integral to the concept of a natural body, meant that some dancers achieved agency at the ideological expense of others. This problem was particularly evident in the experience of members of the British company Phoenix, whose cultural heritage was displaced. Through funding requirements, government agencies and other institutions imposed artistic approaches associated with Somatics because they signified creative authenticity, thereby exploiting dancers who embraced Somatics.

In my own efforts to find a way forward as a longtime practitioner and believer in the power and efficacy of Somatics training, I have endeavored to integrate into my teaching the understanding that, rather than unearthing natural movement, dancers construct nature to achieve a sense of authenticity against what they experience as imposed aesthetics. As part of studio classes, I have tried to teach students to reflect on how ideas of collectivism and individuality are synthesized through Somatics using the rhetoric of natural capacity. The consciousness I brought to teaching helped me refrain from imposing aesthetics that I associated with the conceit of authenticity. Initially in classes not based on set movement, I had perceived students as failing to transcend "imposed aesthetics" when they embodied Somatics through vocabulary familiar to them. I wanted them to "let go" of what they knew, but, cognizant of the insights in my study, I realized I was looking for pedestrian-like forms, particular timing, and other aesthetics. Apparently I needed to "let go" of my preconceptions about "authenticity" to allow the students to use aesthetics that they valued. They asserted movement ideas that pushed against my more homogenized aesthetic. One student described bringing the skills learned in my classes to hip-hop, which alerted me to my assumption that he would bring hip-hop to contemporary dance—the dominant idiom in the dance program where I was teaching, as it is in most other American university dance programs. The student contested contemporary dance's superiority by insisting upon his autonomy over the Somatics skills he was learning, which bolstered my belief in the potential use of the regimens to critique the homogenization of technique and vocabulary.

Using this adaptability of Somatics modalities to different vocabularies, I also choreographed work that draws attention to how contemporary dance excludes disabled dancers. The British dancer Catherine Long cannot access most training because of her difference from what is assumed to be a normal bodily structure. Yet using Somatics, I developed with her a vocabulary based on her physicality, a vocabulary that critiqued the aesthetics by which she is generally excluded. Compared with nondisabled people, Long is invariably represented as lacking the capability to do everyday activity properly, such as walking or balancing. Unlike most dance techniques, many Somatics exercises, particularly those associated with the 1970s and those focused on idiosyncratic movement that 1980s East Village artists used, do not depend on the presumption of a normative physical structure. I adapted these approaches to train Long while developing movement that critiqued exclusionary aesthetics. The 2014 solo *Impasse* emphasized the awkwardness and incapability with which Long's movement is usually associated. The dance conveyed the experience of debilitation or paralysis that Long often associates with being visible as a moving body. Yet by executing the dance with physical capacity she cultivated using Somatics, Long exercised agency over the effects of how she is generally represented. Ideas that have been important in Somatics, such as physical autonomy and the critique of established skills, therefore underpinned the creation of choreography that highlighted how contemporary dance reifies a particular idea of physical ability. Rather than stage a physical natural truth, *Impasse* announced the symbolic role of movement in differentiating bodies as elegant and capacious or awkward and incapacitated.

My choreographic critique of elegance and capacity in *Impasse* and my student's use of the regimens in hip-hop both participate in cultural dissidence. Like many scholars and artists, I am invested in the contemporary moving body as a site at which marginalization can be contested along axes such as race, ethnicity, gender, sexuality, and dis/ability. Over the last forty years, Somatics has underpinned much of the methodology by which dance artists have contested misrepresentation or cultivated vocabulary that stages new social subjects. Yet, as I have argued, this traps them in a double bind, because as they assert an authentic self against dominant oppressive ideals, they also extend neoliberal ideology by staging cultural dissidence as proof of their creative and social freedom. Even if dancers refer to existing vocabulary in their choreography, Somatics still configures the body as a tabula rasa at the point of training, through which various traditions can be embodied to launch critical projects. Scholars who theorize that Somatics informed dance as a contestation of prevailing and oppressive ideals similarly recapitulate the idealization of cultural dissidence in liberal capitalism. Somatics-based dance claims to provide freedom from establishment constraints and the space to stage critique, but in a way that allows liberalism to sidestep interrogation by seeming to be the basis from which critique is possible.

By describing my implementation of Somatics, I want to stress that although accessing natural physical capacity does not guarantee dancers' agency, we can, through our teaching and choreography, become attuned to the social, political, cultural, and economic processes of subjugation. Of course, some artists, particularly those associated with the British 1970s collective X6, and East Village artists beginning in the 1980s, took note of the body's sociopolitical relevance. Yet their uses of the training continued to invest in the idea of nature, with which they cultivated distinct Somatics bodies to negotiate different circumstances. Because practitioners invariably believed that they were pursuing authenticity that is integral to the natural body, the causes of the tensions that arose with the diversification of pedagogy and choreography were overshadowed. Further research would reveal whether this pursuit of authenticity ultimately robbed artists of a language to challenge the effects of institutionalization or if they found ways within Somatics discourse to continue their resistance. Toward the end of the twentieth century, dance training programs and concert houses began asserting their belief in artistic freedom by engaging both highly successful and more marginal artists who seemed to share a pedagogical and artistic heritage to which Somatics was integral. They embraced well-known choreographers who guaranteed large audiences and promised students access to the knowledge required to join a company. The institutions also, however, included marginal artists who would be appreciated by well-informed dance audiences and teach students about innovation. A shared discourse, that the artists were experimenting with natural physical capacity, concealed the material and cultural conditions that mediated the choices artists were able to make. If, however, we understand the search for authenticity as the pursuit of agency against myriad forms subjugation, as well as the capitalizing upon of available opportunities, then the question becomes not what is the right way to access natural physical capacity, but how do dancers contend with their circumstances?

The widespread shift in the twenty-first century toward using Somatics as a complement to classic training calls for an investigation of how the values in the regimens have changed to support the execution of existing vocabulary as opposed to training dancers to generate their own styles. The broad institutionalization of Somatics happened at a time when dance education began embodying a competitive corporate model. But with my focus on the rapid growth and then decline of a community identified with experimentation, this study neglects to analyze the values constructed in the studio by dancers who aim to cultivate excellence in the execution of existing vocabularies, including ballet and modern dance. What I did uncover was that some institutions changed their use of Somatics from cultivating idiosyncratic dancers to promoting the regimens as a way to protect health and enjoy career longevity. But finding out more about how the language of the practice changed will reveal how the use of Somatics as a source of innovation in the late twentieth century relates to its use as a source of excellence in execution in twenty-first-century dance education. I would ask whether or not the principles established in the period from the 1960s to the 1990s continue to be asserted as the foundation of the work.

Along with the questions about how Somatics reconfigures itself in relation to non-Western dance forms and in non-Western contexts, the further research I am proposing calls for a substantial focus on major dance training institutions. The Singapore Dance Academy, P.A.R.T.S. in Belgium (which is thought to be at the cutting edge of contemporary dance training), Julliard (which remains the most well-known conservatory for dancers in the United States), and the London School of Contemporary Dance all figure as major institutions in different countries that look to a transnational context for contemporary dance. These institutions also all implement Somatics in their effort to establish a competitive edge in the dance education market. The question becomes, then: how do teachers and students use the idea of authenticity and its undergirding conception of the natural in these contexts, where the aim is clearly not to resist dance establishments, but to achieve success within them?

Brief Biographies of Some Key Somatics Practitioners

Alexander, Fredrick Matthias. Founder of the Alexander Technique, Alexander was an actor and teacher born in 1869 in Tasmania, Australia. While experimenting with head and neck positioning to find a solution for his chronic laryngitis, Alexander became aware of habitual movements that were hindering his expression and quality of voice. He developed the Alexander Technique in the latter part of the nineteenth century, taught it in Melbourne and Sydney, and eventually brought his method to London and New York. Over the course of his lifetime, Alexander further developed the technique to assist and aid others, primarily individuals in the performing arts, in overcoming their dysfunction and using their bodies better as a whole. Alexander believed that the dynamic relationship between the head, neck, and spine was crucial to a person's overall well-being. He referred to this as primary control. He stressed the importance of inhibition to alter routine movement. He postulated that by stopping a movement from occurring, one could rest the action and redirect motion to function more "naturally." Over time, as movements reset, they can be expected to become second nature, and the result may include an array of different effects, including improvement of movement, posture, or voice quality and decrease of physical pain. The technique thus is a method of re-educating people in how they use themselves (efficiently) in ordinary activities of daily life like walking, sitting, and standing, as well as extraordinary activities such as singing, dancing, and playing sports, with the goal to create more ease and freedom from strain.

Bainbridge Cohen, Bonnie. Bainbridge Cohen is a movement artist, researcher, educator, and occupational therapist. She received a BS in Occupational Therapy from The Ohio State University, where she also studied dance, and she also studied Laban Movement Analysis at the Laban/Bartenieff Institute of Movement Studies. Her teachers included Barbara Clark and André Bernard (Clark is a protégé of Mabel Todd, who is one of the first pioneers of Somatics education, and Bernard was Clark's student); Yogi Ramira in yoga; and Haruchi Noguchi in Japan, founder of Katsugen Undo, a method of training the involuntary nervous systems. Bainbridge Cohen began her research in movement therapy and experiential anatomy in 1958, which eventually led her to establish a system she calls "Body-Mind Centering (BMC)" Within the system of BMC, movement is used as a medium to observe the expressions of the mind through the body and as a way to effect changes in the body/mind relationship. A central aspect in the process of BMC is aligning the inner cellular movement with the external manifestation of movement through space. There are many ways of working toward this alignment, such as through touch, movement, visualization, vocalization, music, and meditation. The process of alignment involves identifying, articulating, differentiating, and integrating the various tissues within the body and discovering the qualities they contribute to one's movement efficiency. The study of BMC includes both the cognitive and experiential learning of the body systems—skeleton, ligaments, muscles, fascia, fat, skin, organs, endocrine glands, nerves, and fluids; breathing and vocalization; the senses and the dynamics of perception; developmental movement; and psychophysical integration. Bainbridge Cohen established The School for Body-Mind Centering in 1973.

Bernard, André. Born in 1924 in Columbia, South Carolina, Bernard pursued majors in chemistry and mathematics. He also enrolled in courses in the arts toward the end of his college years and developed an interest in theater, later becoming a dancer in the Erick Hawkins Dance Company. Bernard developed an interest in Ideokinesis in pursuit of an acting career. He was trained by Barbara Clark in a "physio-philosophical" approach to movement, and he later became an anatomy teacher incorporating embodied functional movement lessons for dancers. At the time that Bernard became a student of Clark in the 1950s, Mabel Todd's prominence in New York was waning. Concerned that the work would be lost when Todd closed her New York studio, Clark, with the help of Bernard and Joanne Emmons, formed an organization devoted to the continuance of the teaching that she called the "Technique of Movement." Bernard's work in body alignment harmonized beautifully with his study of acting at Drama Tree, the school of Anthony Mannino. Mannino trained actors in the Meisner Technique, which was based on the original theories of the Russian director Konstantin Stanislavsky. The year 1965 also brought Bernard the opportunity to teach alignment classes for the Dance Department at the Tisch School for the Arts. In 1970 his appointment broadened to include the Dance Division of the School of Education, Health, Nursing and Arts Professions at New York University (NYU). At NYU, Bernard enlarged the scope of his classes, which included lectures on the scientific aspects of the field based in the works of Mabel Todd and Lulu Sweigard.

Clark, Barbara. Barbara Clark was first a client and then a student of Todd's. She wrote three manuals for coaching more efficient movement, *Let's Enjoy Sitting-Standing-Walking* (1963), *How to Live in Your Axis—Your Vertical Line* (1968), and *Body Proportion Needs Depth* (1975), that are roughly suggestive of her approach. A highly respected and sought-after teacher, Clark mentored André Bernard, John Rolland, Nancy Topf, Marsha Paludan, Mary Fulkerson, and other formative figures in Somatics pedagogy. She also worked with infants and schoolchildren as well as dancers and actors to impart a sense of neuromuscular alignment. As the most direct source for understanding Todd's approach, she influenced generations of Somatics practitioners.

De Groot, Pauline. As a dancer, choreographer, and teacher from the Netherlands, De Groot was an influential figure in the New Dance circuit in North America and Europe in the 1960s. Her early training and performance experience in the United States with Martha Graham, José Limón, Merce Cunningham, Erick Hawkins, and André Bernard established her kinship with the "Judson Church generation" and her rooting in the American avant-garde. She integrated into her work principles of movement disciplines such as Tai Chi, Chi Kung, Todd Alignment, Alexander Technique, release technique, Contact Improvisation, martial arts, and yoga, as well as the teachings of Buddha. On her return to the Netherlands in 1965, introducing new ideas about movement and aesthetics, De Groot founded a school in her studio that later formed the foundation of the School for New Dance Development (SNDD) (1976) of the Amsterdam School of Higher Education in the Arts. As one of the main teachers at the SNDD for twenty years, De Groot was influential to several generations of dancers and makers in the field today. The performance of improvisation is essential in DeGroot's work. In her teaching she calls for an engagement with the senses that clarifies, supports, and energizes the body and the mind into performance, vitality, and well-being.

Dowd, Irene. Dowd majored in philosophy at Vassar College, where she completed a thesis on body image in relation to movement for her Bachelor of Arts degree. After graduating from Vassar in 1968, she was accepted into the Julliard School, Dance Division as a special studies student focusing on choreography, and it is here that she became a student and then assistant of Lulu Sweigard. During her six years of intensive study with Sweigard, learning functional anatomy for dancers and Sweigard's approach to individual instruction in ideokinetic facilitation, Dowd also undertook the study of human anatomy and neuroanatomy at Columbia Presbyterian Medical School. Along with Sweigard, she implemented the interpretation of Todd's work to support ballet and modern training at Julliard. Having studied dance with Cunningham, Lucas Hoving, Antony Tudor, and Viola Farber, among others, she also became a student of the movement sciences, exploring the areas of motor control, brain lateralization, motor development, sensory and motor integration, the neurobehavioral basis of locomotion, biomechanics, and individualized fitness training. Her book *Taking Root to Fly* was highly influential within the Somatics community.

Fulkerson, Mary. Mary Fulkerson is a dancer and choreographer originally from the United States where she received a BFA and MFA from the University of Illinois, experimenting with release techniques with her colleagues, Joan Skinner and Marsha Paludan. In addition to collaborations with Skinner and Paludan, Fulkerson also developed further the principles and practices of Ideokinesis by Mabel Todd, Barbara Clark, and Lulu Sweigard in order to establish her own approach to expressive human movement called "Anatomical Release Technique" (ART). The three major concerns of ART include the anatomical, the kinetic, and choreography. Similar to other release techniques, Fulkerson's teaching method emphasized alignment, concentration, focus, a close investigation of one's thought process, and an active integration of mind and body. Deriving from and further developing Todd's detailed studies of optimal anatomical alignment and function—methods that utilized mental imagery within the body to facilitate improvement of posture and ease of movement—Fulkerson devised approaches in service of supporting and inspiring creative movement that flowed through a well-aligned and easeful body. Fulkerson evolved her main teachings at the Dartington College of Arts (United Kingdom) between 1973 and 1985, during which time she advocated an approach where physical presence, full embodiment, and body-mind centering could provide students ways to generate personal vocabularies alongside their training in classical and modern dance. The dance department at Dartington, under her leadership, was critical to the evolution of New Dance in the United Kingdom in the 1970s and 1980s, and more widely across Europe. She then went on to teach in the Netherlands at the European Dance Development Center (EDDC).

Hassall, Nanette. Choreographer, dancer, and teacher Nanette Hassall was born in Sydney, Australia, where she received her early training at the Bodenwieser Centre. Traveling to the United States, she graduated from Julliard in 1969 and subsequently danced with the Merce Cunningham Company while also attending many of the experimental dance performances in New York. In 1973, she moved to London, where she performed, choreographed, and taught for Ballet Rambert and Strider. Returning to Sydney in 1975, she joined Jaap Flier's Dance Company and then, with Russell Dumas, founded Dance Exchange. In 1983, she moved to Melbourne, where she founded Dance Works and continued to choreograph numerous works for this company. Throughout her time with Dance Exchange and Dance Works and in her subsequent teaching at the Western Australia Academy of Performing Arts, Hassall introduced a range of Somatics approaches to dance students and encouraged exchange with other Somatics-oriented institutions abroad. She retired as head of the Dance Department at Western Australia in 2019.

H'Doubler, Margaret. Considered to be a pioneer for American dance in higher education, H' Doubler was born in Kansas in 1889. She studied biology at the University of Wisconsin, and after her graduation in 1910, she was asked to stay and teach in the Department of Physical

Education for women. Subsequently attending graduate school at Columbia University, she developed new ideas about the subject of dance in higher education and upon her return began an approach to dance that involved both the body and the mind. Her amalgam of open-ended dance explorations on the floor coupled with the study of biological sciences became requisite studies within the first university dance department at the University of Wisconsin, where she established the first dance major in higher education in 1926 within the Department of Physical Education. She laid out her approach to dance education in the 1921 text *A Manual of Dancing*. During her career H'Doubler rejected notions of educational dance as professionally focused "art-dance" in favor of the more liberal idea of dance as the creative side of movement. She strived to keep dancing a liberal and nonstratified, creative learning experience, one that was especially beneficial to women, who were exposed to radical new ways to explore and understand their bodies. Her focus on exploration in dance as distinct from imitation endured throughout the twentieth century in the rhetoric of university programs that privilege investigation and understanding above success and competition in professional dance.

Karczag, Eva. Karczag has been an advocate for explorative methods of dance making since the early 1970s, and her performance work and teaching are informed by dance improvisation and mindful body practices including the Alexander Technique and Ideokinesis. She received an MFA degree from Bennington College and has taught dance at major colleges and studios throughout the United States, Australia, and Europe, including a sustained period of teaching on the faculty of the EDDC in Arnhem, Netherlands, from 1990 to 2002. Karczag improvises resistance toward the institutional appropriation of a Somatics approach. In Somatics training and related choreographic modalities, she cultivates principles of physical ease and individual authenticity. She brought this facility to the development of some of Trisha Brown's signature works when she joined the company in 1979, yet she left in 1985 because she was concerned that New York's careerist arts culture was erasing her creative uniqueness. Since 1985, she has pursued improvisation and experimentation on the margins of Euro-American contemporary dance, while resisting commercial ideas of innovation. Her Somatics approach insists that dancers cultivate optimum capacity for movement execution, providing unlimited resources for creativity by accessing the body's anatomical functional imperatives.

Klein, Susan. A former dancer and movement therapist, Klein created a movement education system in collaboration with her partner Barbara Mahler, eventually called the Klein Technique. One of its central goals was minimization of risk of injury among dancers. The technique is a clinical practice constructed using basic principles of physics and anatomy, and borrows and builds upon theories and exercises from Bartenieff Fundamentals, Laban Movement Analysis, Worsley Five-Element Acupuncture, and Zero Balancing. One of the most significant influences that Bartenieff had on Klein was her application of "thrust and counterthrust." Bartenieff believed that without a kinesthetic understanding of this concept, dancers could jeopardize their "connection" or relationship to space and the ground. Klein further argued that it was a loss of this connection that was the root cause of many musculoskeletal injuries. The Klein Technique offers dancers a theoretical and practical underpinning, independent of choreographic style or aesthetic agenda, to negotiate the forces of gravity through the skeletal system in order to improve technique, athleticism, and virtuosity and to heal and prevent injury. Klein taught dancers how to repattern unproductive movement habits by working at what she calls the "level of the bone," a focus that changed the relationship of the bones to each other, relative to ground and space. In learning the technique, dancers work to align their bones by using the deep muscle groups in the pelvis that are responsible for the transfer of forces through the body—the psoas, the hamstrings (connecting sitz bones to heels), and the pelvic floor—to find the deep support between the tail and the pubic bone and the external rotators. Influencing a host of dancers over many years, Klein first opened her school, the Susan Klein School of Movement and Dance, in downtown Manhattan in 1979.

Paludan, Marsha. As a graduate teaching assistant at the University of Illinois, Paludan, along with Fulkerson, Rolland, Topf, and Skinner, developed collaborative and individual versions of Anatomical Release, cross-pollinating ideas and visions in a process of developing release technique as an alternative dance technique. Early release work was a process of sensory and kinesthetic training and imaging exercises that in her words "freed the imagination in order to free the body." Paludan subsequently studied developmental movement with Barbara Clark. In the 1980s, while pursuing a PhD in Theatre at the University of Kansas, Paludan met Marjorie Barstow and knew immediately that the Alexander Technique was the missing piece to her vast body of work. She apprenticed with her in later years, working together to develop movement education in the US Midwest. From 1991 to 2008, Paludan was a professor of theater at the University of North Carolina at Greensboro, where she coordinated the movement curriculum for both the MFA and BFA acting programs.

Rolland, John. An important figure in the development of release and alignment technique, Rolland met Nancy Topf when he was a student at the University of Illinois in the late 1960s. Topf and Rolland began an intense dialogue exploring concepts that Marsha Paludan and Joan Skinner had started to engage with a few years before as teachers at the same university, which questioned traditional methods of training the body. Subsequently, but at different times, John Rolland, Marsha Paludan, Mary Fulkerson, and Nancy Topf became students of Barbara Clark. It was Clark's work that helped to define the theoretical and technical foundation for much of their own research. Along with Paludan, Fulkerson, and Topf, Rolland established studio procedures for Anatomical Releasing and a movement vocabulary that manifested the idea of divesting dance of aesthetics into a recognizable training system. With Paludan and Topf, Rolland established a workshop in 1976 that came to be known as the Vermont Movement Workshop and lasted for twelve years. They established a curriculum that included Todd alignment work, release technique, Contact Improvisation, and composition classes called "Structures of Improvisation." In 1982, Rolland was invited to become a member of the teaching staff at the Modern Dance Department of the state-run Theatre School in Amsterdam. At the school, Rolland developed and applied a new model of teaching that freed dance training from stylistic limitations yet still conveyed basic technical knowledge.

Skinner, Joan. Joan Skinner is an American choreographer, teacher, improvisation pioneer, and former dancer with the Martha Graham and Merce Cunningham Companies. She developed an innovative approach to dance and movement in the early 1960s called Skinner Releasing Technique (SRT) while serving as the chair of the Dance Department at the University of Washington. To develop her technique, she applied her own experiences of dancing, principles of alignment and movement that she encountered while studying Alexander Technique, and work on imagination and visualization by Mabel Todd. SRT can be described as a system of kinesthetic training that refines the perception and performance of movement through the use of imagery utilizing image-guided floorwork to ease tension and promote an effortless kind of moving, integrated with alignment of the whole self. Tactile exercises are used to give the imagery immediate kinesthetic effect. A person practicing SRT ideally lets go of habitual holding patterns and ways of thinking in order to let something new happen, discover natural alignment, and thereby improve not only strength and flexibility but also access new kinds of spontaneity and creativity. Throughout the 1970s, SRT was taught by Skinner and the American

Contemporary Dance Company, primarily in Seattle, and the work continues to be taught and practiced today, deeply influencing many contemporary movement artists. The four principles of SRT are multidirectional skeletal alignment, multidirectional balancing, autonomy of breath and movement, and economy of movement (only using the necessary muscles with a minimum expenditure of energy).

Starks Whitehouse, Mary. A West Coast pioneer of dance therapy (based in Los Angeles), Mary Stark Whitehouse began the work she called "movement in depth" in the 1950s. Based on her dance training with Mary Wigman and Jungian psychoanalysis, Whitehouse developed a rich and detailed movement bridge to inner experience, including the unconscious, direct sensation, dreams, and interpersonal dynamics. The inspiration for Whitehouse to develop this practice occurred in the 1950s when she felt that modern dance had divested the body of its innate capacity for expression with stereotyped vision that manifested through an overinvestment in virtuosity. In her regimen of Authentic Movement, Whitehouse aimed to recuperate individual creativity from the ossification it experienced through routine daily life by releasing the private psychic process in Jungian-based therapy. One of her central principles was the importance of attending to inner experience and moving in dialogue with or response to that rich inner experience. In other words, the core of the movement experience she explored is the sensation of both moving and being moved at the same moment, activated with attention, allowing and following the "authentic" movement impulse.

Sweigard, Lulu. Also considered a pioneer in the work of Ideokinesis, Dr. Lulu Sweigard was a student of Todd's in the later 1920s at Columbia University. Like her mentor, Sweigard emphasized structural alignment, which she called "postural pattern," and she proposed that each individual had one true postural alignment. Sweigard emphasized the scientific aspect of the work Todd had established by conducting empirical research. In 1929, she set out to determine whether Ideokinesis could recoordinate muscle action enough to produce measurable changes in skeletal alignment. She hypothesized that prolonged training in Ideokinesis would lead to specific changes in skeletal alignment, which she went on to prove successfully. She taught the work at NYU from the mid-1930s through the mid-1950s and then went on to teach at the Julliard School of Dance, where she continued until her death. Her findings radically transformed the way people, especially dancers, thought about their bodies because prior to Sweigard, the dominant theory was that weak muscles were the cause of poor posture, and that strengthening these muscles by holding, straightening, and tightening would produce the desired effects. In contrast to these widely accepted practices, Sweigard demonstrated that shifting the focus of movement initiation from body to mind was pivotal as long as an appropriate image was visualized. Without contributing any effort to performing movement, the body could be brought to its correct alignment. Thus, relaxation and the ability to imagine within Sweigard's system became key to attaining an efficient mechanical equilibrium.

Todd, Mabel Elsworth. Author of *The Thinking Body* (1937), Todd, along with Alexander, was one of the first generation of Somatics practitioners. Her approach, named Ideokinesis, employs the use of images as a means of improving muscle patterns. Searching for a means to improve her walking impairment (caused by a paralyzing accident in her youth), she began to develop imagery focused around the anatomically balanced use of the body. During her research, Todd speculated that vocal problems were often due to bad posture and that a psycho-physical or psycho-physiological approach might help. With this hypothesis, Todd began to study the mechanics of the skeletal structure in 1906 at Emerson College (where she was studying voice), and she applied her discoveries in her studios of "Natural Posture" in New York and Boston in the 1920s working primarily as a voice improvement teacher. She focused on achieving a balance between bone and muscle support. According to Todd, movement is more subject to mental pictures than conscious direction. The classic Todd image was the "up the front and down the back of the spine"—wherein "up the front" activates tensile musculature in the front of the spine, and the "release down the back" is intended to release the spine from the muscles in the back so that it can become its own support. Todd joined the faculty of the Department of Physical Education at Teachers College, Columbia University, where she taught anatomy, posture, and neuromuscular awareness to physical education and dance professionals.

Topf, Nancy. Choreographer, dancer, and teacher, Nancy Topf was a graduate of the University of Wisconsin. She received her primary training from Merce Cunningham and Barbara Clark and also studied with Robert Joffrey, Anna Halprin, and Steve Paxton. Topf was a pioneer in the areas of bodywork, release technique, and dance improvisation. Living in New York City since the mid-1960s and then teaching at the University of Illinois in the early 1970s, she participated in the beginnings of release and Contact Improvisation, working with dancers such as Steve Paxton, Joan Skinner, Marsha Paludan, and Mary Fulkerson, eventually finding in Barbara Clark's work the knowledge that inspired her approach. While Todd's approach was deeply founded in anatomical imagery, Topf became known for honing in on the importance of the center of the body and the work of the psoas in efficient human expression. Topf developed a technique of neuromuscular retraining, which involved a repatterning and realignment of the body that many dancers found helpful for healing chronic injuries and focusing on their creative work. From Topf's point of view, release work evolved simultaneously with Contact Improvisation. She felt that many aspects united these two forms of movement, for example, an interest in the creative process, improvisation, experimentation, exploration, and a redefining of the use of the body and weight.

Notes

Introduction

1. The regimens on which I focus include Body-Mind Centering, Skinner Releasing Technique, Anatomical Release, Authentic Movement, Klein Technique, and Contact Improvisation. Although some might convincingly argue that Contact Improvisation is a very separate practice, I hope to show that its early development was deeply entwined with the other practices, and that even in their distinctive forms, they developed through interaction with each other.
2. In his study of Graham's career, Mark Franko shows how her work overall is regularly reduced to the meaning that it accrued in the 1970s. However, the fact that by the 1970s Graham's dancers were taking ballet classes, and in line with the culture of ballet they were attempting to emulate the style of the choreographer, contributes to understanding the way that dancers experimenting with Somatics distinguished themselves from modern dance. Mark Franko, *Dancing Modernism/Performing Politics* (Bloomington: Indiana University Press, 1995), 50.
3. Although I focus on only six techniques, they by no means represent the comprehensive field of Somatics. Feldenkrais has increasingly become important for dancers, and Kinetic Awareness Work had an enormous impact in the 1960s and 1970s on the adoption of a particular way the body moves in concert dance through Trisha Brown's choreography. However, the six techniques on which I focus became practices around which dancers formed particularly strong alliances in the historical period that my study covers. Furthermore, the physical and textual metaphors developed for the body in the six techniques seem to have penetrated dancers' studio practice to a greater degree than have other Somatics approaches.
4. In his PhD dissertation, "Surface to Essence: Appropriation of the Orient by Modern Dance," Mark Wheeler withholds critique of the appropriation of what he calls Eastern ideas and aesthetics undertaken by white American artists. He asserts that CI and Body-Mind Centering manifest the deepest truths of non-Western ideas. Mark Wheeler, "Surface to Essence: Appropriation of the Orient by Modern Dance" (PhD diss., University of Illinois, 1984). In contrast, I apply Edward Said's observation in *Orientalism* that bifurcating global regions into essential cultural differences is reductive and misrepresentative. This is the manner in which white artists achieve their apparent neutrality. The avant-garde, therefore, affords the Oriental contemporary relevance and legibility while excluding the non-Western subject, a subject that is marked as ancient and culturally specific against the newly constructed "neutral" body of the white artist. Edward Said, *Orientalism* (New York: Pantheon Books, 1978).
5. Dixon Gottschild argues that Africanist movement aesthetics were assimilated into Europeanist avant-garde choreographic approaches. The relaxed body of the postmodern dancer and the use of pedestrian movement, for example, were initially cultivated,

sustained, and transferred through African American jazz and tap dance lineages, but then appeared in Judson and other white avant-garde experiments. Brenda Dixon Gottschild, *Digging the Africanist Presence in American Performance: Dance and Other Contexts, Contributions in Afro-American and African Studies* (Westport, CT: Greenwood Press, 1996). At the same time, Somatics pedagogy often relied on the metaphors referencing the primitive. Skinner Releasing, for example, uses the term "animal quality" to describe a reconnection with nature.

6. Morris explains that by rejecting explicit themes, Cunningham avoided McCarthy-led government intrusiveness while also circumnavigating a perceived threat to modern dance's artistic pedigree from commercialism. Gay Morris, *A Game for Dancers: Performing Modernism in the Postwar Years, 1945–1960* (Middletown, CT: Wesleyan University Press, 2006), 174.

7. Among other scholars who argue for the role axes of identity in social change, I draw on the work of Linda Tomko in *Dancing Class: Gender, Ethnicity, and Social Divides in American Dance, 1890–1920*. Tomko points out that by constructing universal themes staged in the Lower East Side at Settlement House festivals, middle-class, Jewish women attempted to gloss class differences and smooth over anti-Semitism exhibited toward working-class recent immigrant Jews. Linda J. Tomko, *Dancing Class: Gender, Ethnicity, and Social Divides in American Dance, 1890–1920* (Bloomington: Indiana University Press, 1999), 81. Similarly to Morris, Rebekah Kowal insists that race must be understood as a factor in the work of Merce Cunningham in her *How to Do Things with Dance: Performing Change in Postwar America* (Middletown, CT: Wesleyan University Press, 2010), 186.

8. Cynthia Jean Cohen-Bull, "Sense Meaning and Perception in Three Dance Cultures," in *Meaning in Motion: New Cultural Studies of Dance*, ed. Jane Desmond (Durham, NC: Duke University Press, 1997), 271.

9. Ibid., 285.

10. For example, she focused less on the specificity of sense and perception and more on how they functioned in the antihierarchical communitarian value system of CI. Yet, based on such abstraction, she was able to track the hostility that arose within the community when a hierarchy seemed to emerge. Some dancers distinguished themselves as teachers and performers by deploying the sensual and perceptive skills associated with physical cooperation for purposes of virtuoso display. Cynthia J. Novack, *Sharing the Dance: Contact Improvisation and American Culture* (Madison: University of Wisconsin Press, 1990), 221.

11. For example, Jon McKenzie reviews late twentieth-century theories of management that increase efficiency by shifting from "top-down" decision making to diffuse responsibility. Jon McKenzie, *Perform or Else: From Discipline to Performance* (London: Routledge, 2001), 55–95.

12. See, for example, Pamela Matt, *A Kinesthetic Legacy: The Life and Works of Barbara Clark* (Tempe, AZ: CMT Press, 1993) or the chapbook arranged by Melinda Buckwalter, "The Anatomy of Center by Nancy Topf," *Contact Quarterly Chapbook 3* 37, no. 2 (Summer/Fall 2012).

13. See, for example, Rebecca Nettl-Fiol and Luc Vanier, *Dance and the Alexander Technique: Exploring the Missing Link* (Urbana, IL: University of Chicago Press, 2011).

Chapter 1

1. Leslie Kaminoff, "Release," *Movement Research Performance Journal* 18 (Winter/Spring 1999): 1.
2. He argued that "man" moved beyond purely instinctual imperatives, such as natural selection, by evolving consciousness, but that various "natural" dimensions of the body still needed to be brought under conscious control, which could be done through his regimen.
3. Frederick Matthias Alexander, *Man's Supreme Inheritance* (New York: E. P. Dutton & Company, 1918).
4. Ibid., 6.
5. Ibid., 72.
6. Alexander himself actually universalized his theory in texts such as *The Use of the Self: Its Conscious Direction in Relation to Diagnosis, Functioning and the Control of Reaction* (New York: E. P. Dutton & Co., 1932). It is notable that this text was published in the 1930s, a full twenty years after the racial theories in *Man's Supreme Inheritance*.

    Dewey wrote the introduction to several of Alexander's books, including *Man's Supreme Inheritance* (1918), *Constructive Conscious Control of the Individual* (1923), *The Use of the Self* (1932), and *A Universal Constant in Living* (1941). Alexander began teaching Dewey at Columbia University in 1915, and they sustained a professional relationship for forty years, including Dewey writing the forward for Alexander's work and professing the value of his technique publicly. Alexander was also connected to other intellectuals within the progressive education movement through his work at Columbia University (Michael Huxley. "F. Matthias Alexander and Mabel Elsworth Todd: Proximities, Practices and the Psycho-Physical." *Journal of Dance and Somatic Practices* 3, nos. 1–2 (2012): 27.

    The mutually influencing relationship between Alexander and Dewey has not received the attention it deserves, in terms of how their respective work may be indebted to each other's ideas. Yet, the importance of Alexander's and Dewey's ideas for each other is documented. See, for example, a series of booklets, edited by Alexander Murray, *John Dewey and F.M. Alexander* (Dayton, OH: AmSAT Books, 1991–92).
7. Alexander called for education that worked with the body and reordered consciousness such that the natural propensities tied to the evolutionary process could be corralled by bringing them under conscious control. In turn, Dewey contributed the idea of embodied reflection to education, which emerged through his relationship to Alexander.
8. Fallace explains that the two dominant evolutionary ideas both presumed an inherent capacity of life forms: the materialist that early forms are superior and the idealist that the opposite is the case. Dewey argued that difference is due to social context, not biologically determined capacity, which underpinned his progressive views on racial difference. Thomas D. Fallace, "Was John Dewey Ethnocentric? Reevaluating the Philosopher's Early Views on Culture and Race," *Educational Researcher* 39, no. 6 (2010): 474.
9. Dewey certainly stratified culture in a teleology of Western superiority through his belief in "linear historicism," but he challenged biological racism and class superiority by arguing that the "savage" is evident in the "civilized," and environment determines intellectual capacity. Ibid.
10. Dewey argued that learning follows natural stages that reflect individual psychological as well as sociological development. Corporeality was seen to be key to learning because, like Alexander, Dewey felt that education entailed resolving the instinctual dimensions of

human beings with the rational. Consequently, Dewey posed a challenge for entrenched nineteenth-century ideas about education by taking recourse to the agency of the body, to which cultural stratification was integral. For a deeper consideration of the ways in which Dewey's work has been configured in relation to racial theories in the early twentieth century, see Fallace, "Was John Dewey Ethnocentric?"

11. Gelb's book is peppered with images of African tribespeople, animals, and children, accompanied with captions such as this one: "The natural dignity of this Nuba tribesman is expressed in his upright stature and the poise of his head." Gelb, *Body Learning*, 55.

12. Alexander argues that posture is a universal constant and source for salvation in human experience, which he articulated in his 1941 text, *The Universal Constant in Living*. Michael Huxley, "F. Matthias Alexander and Mabel Elsworth Todd: Proximities, Practices and the Psycho-Physical," *Journal of Dance and Somatic Practices* 3, nos. 1–2 (2012): 30.

13. Janice Ross gives a clear description of Dewey's perspective on education relative to various dualisms and the way that H'Doubler cultivated a dance educational approach based on his theories in her chapter, "Margaret H'Doubler and the Philosophy of John Dewey," in *Moving Lessons: Margaret H'Doubler and the Beginning of Dance in American Education* (Madison: University of Wisconsin Press, 2000), 124–33.

14. Margaret H'Doubler came into contact with these ideas through Dewey and Alexander, with whom she took lessons. In her writing, H'Doubler referenced both Alexander and Dewey, whose ideas had an enormous impact on an approach to dance education she developed, which was built upon many of the ideas that became central to Somatics practice. Drawing together several texts, including the writing about H'Doubler by Janice Ross, Huxley argues that Alexander had both direct and indirect influence on the dance educationalist. "F. Matthias Alexander," 31.

15. H'Doubler used an exercise in which one partner pulls another partner by their leg when they are relaxed on the floor and twists them completely over by having each part of the body successively respond in the twist. This is a way in which the students could find out how much energy it took for the twist to happen, how much they could relax within the twist, ideas of initiation, and follow-through. She learned this from the children's dance classes she observed in New York. Ross, *Moving Lessons*, 155.

16. For example, she recuperated the skeleton from Victorian iconography where it signified the supposed fatal and infective dangers of immoral social dancing. Ibid., 154.

17. Ross, *Moving Lessons*, 13.

18. Janice Ross argues that the social position of women was central to H'Doubler's project. Ibid., 12. Her analysis aligns with several texts covering the late nineteenth century to the 1930s and suggests that modern dance became a means for women to push beyond separate spheres of ideology in which they were confined to domesticity and also to forge a uniquely feminine subjectivity in the public sphere. See, for example, Ann Daly, *Done into Dance: Isadora Duncan in America* (Bloomington: Indiana University Press, 1995); Franko, *Dancing Modernism*; and Tomko, *Dancing Class*. Ross further argues that H'Doubler's rhetoric paralleled that of Duncan because she gained access for white middle-class women to higher education through the dancing body by distinguishing her approach from African and Spanish American traditions. Ross, *Moving Lessons*, 154. H'Doubler also participated in the class bias of the "new morality," which underpinned her project. Tomko points out that Progressive Era bodies were constructed through the assumption

of sedentary middle-class lifestyles versus the laboring working class. While Delsarte's movement system was thought to be suited to the middle class, educationalists believed the vigorous activity of gross motor movements in folk dance expended excess energy of the working classes, who were infantilized as an overenergetic mass needing to let off steam. They believed working people would not understand the value of improving comportment and, as such, folk dance was a way to disguise the introduction of physical vitality and postural health. Tomko's findings suggest the history of class distinction in the genteel tradition persisted as working people were assumed to not care about posture. *Dancing Class*, 172–73.

19. The term "Ideokinesis" was actually coined by a student and acolyte of Todd, Lulu Sweigard, who published her own text, *Human Movement Potential: Its Ideokinetic Facilitation* (Lanham, MD: University Press of America, 1988), which has become as important for dancers as Todd's text. When I use the term "blueprint," I am not suggesting that the ideas I associate with Todd's contribution can all be traced to her as the originating author. As with Alexander, it is true that her work has been enormously influential in the field, but practitioners such as Forti, who began working with these ideas through Halprin, were not initially influenced by a lineage that is traceable to Todd. Rather, I am arguing that Todd's text is a vivid example of a way of thinking about the body that became central for Somatics.

20. The emphasis on kinesthesia both connects H'Doubler's and Todd's project to Alexander and distinguishes it. Working with sensation and imagery, and even skeletal information, is something that Alexander decidedly did not do. Yet, at the same time, the work with kinesthesia and imagery, in particular, connects Todd's work with Alexander because it marks the way in which she insists that her approach is not about physicality but about thinking; this is the way in which it is distinguished as being about thinking. Huxley, "F. Matthias Alexander," 34.

21. There is no evidence Todd connected with Alexander or H'Doubler, yet all three worked in the same New York milieu and likely influenced one another. Huxley points out that 1990s and early twenty-first-century writing draws links between Todd's and Alexander's work, despite the lack of evidence for a direct connection. He provides evidence of the likelihood that they were aware of each other's work by tracing their geographical proximity and evidence that they were moving in the same intellectual culture, teaching in the same institutions, influencing some of the same people, and using similar ideas. This was the same intellectual culture within which H'Doubler was influenced by Alexander and Dewey. H'Doubler may not have referenced Todd because she was aligned with Dewey and Alexander, and there are suggestions that there was some intellectual disagreement about whether Todd's or Alexander's work was more valid because their techniques were being taught and debated in the same context. Ibid., 28–30.

22. Todd distinguishes her technique from late nineteenth-century body culture by arguing that her concern is with thinking, not exercise regimens. This emphasizes the notion of corporeal consciousness. Ibid., 17.

23. Huxley points out that Todd's emphasis on science differentiates her from Alexander, but that Dewey uses his forward to Alexander's *The Use of the Self* to verify the scientific rigor of Alexander's methods. Ibid., 139. John Rolland suggests that in *The Thinking Body*, Todd attempts to be more academic than in her earlier writing because she was teaching

at a university for the first time when it was written. John Rolland and Jacques Van Eijden, "Alignment and Release: History and Methods," in *Talk, 1982–2006: School for New Dance Development Publication: Dancers Talking about Dance, 15 Interviews and Articles from 3 Decades of Dance Research in Amsterdam,* ed. Jeroen Fabius (Amsterdam: International Theatre & Film Books, 2009), 119.

24. Todd proposes that the form of the body follows a functional imperative. She argues that the systems and components of the body each contribute distinctively to the organism's negotiation of universal forces such as gravity and inertia, and she analyzes anatomical structure using principles of mechanics. So, for example, she details how different systems manage gravitational pull. Bones are configured as the weight-bearing, "compression" members of the body, and muscle and fascia as weight-transferring and -upholding "tensile" members. Similarly, the substructures of the body are analyzed for how they function mechanically within a localized realm. Todd considers what physical demands are placed upon them. So, the body is constructed in Todd's approach through how it manages stress and pressure as a network of systems and structures fulfilling identifiable functions. Todd's scientific analysis of human physiology is positioned among all the other organisms. This bolsters her natural conception of the body because she argues that every species is negotiating comparable physical forces. Todd argues that difference in the physical structure of each species depends on whether they live in the water or on land, how they eat, breathe, and so on. Mabel Elsworth Todd, *The Thinking Body: A Study of the Balancing Forces of Dynamic Man* (New York: P. B. Hoeber, 1937).

25. Ibid., 218.

26. Ibid., 157.

27. Ibid., 33.

28. For example, the image that pockets on the back of the trousers are moving around the sides to the front is argued to release overworked muscles that result from the "turned out" position of classical ballet, while the image of the folding ankle being door-hinge closing is thought to enhance the natural tendency of that joint. Images are also used in specific movements that are designed to cultivate minimal muscular tension, such as the tail bone being a weight on a plumb line during simple plié exercises in which the dancer bends at the knees and hips but aims to sustain the fullest length of the spine. Lionel Popkin, "(Dancer, Choreographer, Faculty in U.C.L.A. Dance Dept.) Discussion with the Author," interview by Doran George, February 5, 2014. In Todd's natural postural training, students also use the Constructive Rest Position to reduce physical tension, which, as Irene Dowd proposes, brings the body to neutral from where the work of repatterning can most effectively take place. She advises that after achieving neutrality, students are able to track whether they are using excess tension as they progress from stillness into movement. Dowd was a student of Lulu Sweigard, who trained with Todd. Both Dowd and Sweigard credit their work to Todd. Irene Dowd, *Taking Root to Fly: Articles on Functional Anatomy*, 3rd rev. ed. (New York: I. Dowd, 1995).

29. Ross, *Moving Lessons*, 130.

30. Gay Morris convincingly argues that the institutionalization of modern dance first happened in midcentury. Morris, *A Game for Dancers*, xiii. Her argument is supported, in part, by the fact that modern choreographers began to receive state funding for the arts

for the first time through the international touring program, an issue I deal with in greater detail in chapter 2. See Naima Prevots, *Dance for Export: Cultural Diplomacy and the Cold War*, Studies in Dance History (Middletown, CT: Wesleyan University Press, 1998), 11. Morris further argues that by the mid-1940s rejection of the canonized strategies of the previous generation became a necessary maneuver for the new avant-garde. She insists that one of the central principles of aesthetic modernism was independence from the market, and yet at the same time, artists depended on institutional support for the survival of their project. She suggests that the way in which modern dancers began to contend with this contradiction in midcentury was that the avant-garde critiqued aesthetic strategies that preceded them to demonstrate independence from the market represented by institutionalized modern dance. Imitation, on the other hand, would indicate that the dance form had become the handmaiden of the institution and by association the market. Morris, *A Game for Dancers*, xviii.

31. My argument is profoundly influenced by Serge Guilbaut's text, *How New York Stole the Idea of Modern Art: Abstract Expressionism, Freedom, and the Cold War* (Chicago: University of Chicago Press, 1983). Guilbaut relates the emergence of a US-based avant-garde art to a disillusionment with communism and fear of fascism, along with mistrust of commerce. Guilbaut, *How New York Stole the Idea of Modern Art*, 2–3.

32. John Martin references the impact of Todd's work on Humphrey's technique in 1936. Huxley, "F. Matthias Alexander," 13. The use of weight and momentum in Limón technique certainly had an impact on dancers who worked with Somatics in the United Kingdom, such as Janet Smith and Gill Clarke, but may also have impacted Steve Paxton and Pauline De Groot, who danced in Limón's company in the 1950s. Pauline De Groot, "(Choreographer and Educator) in Discussion with the Author," interview by Doran George, September 2, 2012.

33. Novack, *Sharing the Dance*, 31.

34. Ibid., 25.

35. Wheeler, *Surface to Essence*, 41.

36. Novack, *Sharing the Dance*, 31.

37. Bernard reports being sent to Clark by Hawkins in 1949. Pamela Matt, "André Bernard," http://www.ideokinesis.com/dancegen/bernard/bernard.htm. Pauline De Groot, who danced for Hawkins in the 1960s, recalls being sent to Bernard, with whom she felt she went through an excruciating process of letting go of what she had learned in Graham and ballet techniques. De Groot, "Discussion with the Author."

38. See, for example, Mark Wheeler's discussion of Eric Hawkins's understanding of the relationship between Zen Buddhism and Ideokinesis. Wheeler, *Surface to Essence*, 231.

39. Novack, *Sharing the Dance*, 26.

40. Franko argues that in the 1960s Graham was the oldest member of a second generation of modern dancers, and as such, she was represented by the contemporary avant-garde as embodying what he calls "bankrupt emotivism." Franko quotes Rainer from 1966 charging that Graham's work could not be related to "anything outside of theatre, since it was usually dramatic and psychological necessity that determined it." Franko, *Dancing Modernism/ Performing Politics*, 40. He proposes that as Graham's aging body deteriorated, she relied on dramatic expression to replace the virtuoso technical execution evident earlier in her career. He suggests that young dancers emulated Graham's overtly theatrical displays, and

consequently, her work became associated with theatrical artifice in the 1960s by artists such as Rainer. Ibid., 39.

41. June Ekman, who became an important Alexander teacher for Trisha Brown's dancers in the 1980s, notes that dancers with whom she was associated in the 1950s talked about Martha Graham as hating women who were younger than her. They felt her neurosis was embedded in the authoritarian manner in which her classes were taught. June Ekman, "(Alexander Teacher to the N.Y. Dance Community) in Discussion with the Author," interview by Doran George, June 4, 2012. Pauline De Groot, who was instrumental in the introduction of Somatics to the Netherlands, felt she had to unlearn ballet and Graham technique to cultivate a receptive relationship to her body and dancing. De Groot, "Discussion with the Author."

42. Dancers such as Ekman and De Groot were attracted to a movement culture that seemed to give more attention to the health and well-being of the dancer, both in the language of training and in the more "flowing" choreography. Both trained in Hawkins technique, with De Groot dancing for him. Ekman and her colleagues were also attracted to Nikolais's classes, which, under the influence of his teacher, Hanya Holm, were seen as having a more lyrical movement style. De Groot, "Discussion with the Author"; Ekman, "Discussion with the Author."

43. June Ekman recalls Wayne being one of the teachers that she and her colleagues took classes with in the 1950s because he focused on the reduction of bodily tension. Ekman, "Discussion with the Author." Paul Langland writes, "From 1943, Allan Wayne taught steadily until his death in 1978 in New York. His students included Irmgard Bartenieff, Meredith Monk, Yvonne Rainer, and Martine Van Hammel. He developed a unique vision in his dancing and teaching, incorporating yogic breath and energy work into his classes to meld dance and the healing arts in an early and powerful experiential technique." Brendan McCall and Paul Langland, "Body of Work: The Life and Teachings of Allan Wayne," *Contact Quarterly* 23, no. 2 (Summer/Fall 1998): 43–49.

44. June Ekman recounts that 1950s dancers viewed techniques that they saw as punishing to be out of date, and instead, they pursued training they felt was respectful of the dancing body, such as that of Hawkins, Nikolais, and Merle Marsicano, who taught a preparation based on Todd's ideas. Ekman, "Discussion with the Author."

45. Ibid.

46. Morris, *A Game for Dancers*, 176.

47. Nancy Ruyter insists that Stebbins's version of the Delsarte must be understood as peculiar to Stebbins. She argues that there is evidence of the influence of the American interpretations of the Delsarte system on Isadora Duncan, Ted Shawn, and Ruth St. Denis, as well as the European pioneers of modern dance. Nancy Lee Chalfa Ruyter, *The Cultivation of Body and Mind in Nineteenth-Century American Delsartism* (Westport, CT: Greenwood Press, 1999), 107–10.

48. Ibid.

49. Both Charlotte Selver and Carola Speads were students of the German Somatics teacher Elsa Gindler. Gindler pioneered a technique that combined breathing and relaxation and was a student of Hedwig Kallmeyer, who, in turn, had been a student of Stebbins. Elaine Summers and Joan Arnold, *Interview with Elaine Summers*, 2010, New York Public Library for the Performing Arts, transcript and digital sound discs.

50. McCall and Langland, "Body of Work," 43–49.

51. Both Pauline De Groot and June Ekman talk about Hawkins's work as being like a version of Graham technique modulated with Somatics information. De Groot, "Discussion with the Author"; Ekman, "Discussion with the Author."

52. Novack, *Sharing the Dance*, 33.

53. Summers and Arnold, *Interview with Elaine Summers*.

54. Cunningham gave a lecture on Halprin's outdoor deck studio in 1957. Ross, *Experience as Dance*, 106. Hawkins encouraged Pauline De Groot to seek out Halprin when she was in California. De Groot, "Discussion with the Author." June Ekman also recalls that when she moved to San Francisco in the late 1950s, Alwin Nikolais suggested she look up Halprin. Ekman, "Discussion with the Author."

55. Ross, *Experience as Dance*, 135.

56. In her book on H'Doubler, Ross argues that Halprin transformed the teacher's idea of "synchronized awareness" into the 1960s psychological aesthetic of "being present in the moment." *Moving Lessons*, 157. Ross details Halprin's use of such ideas in the 1950s. *Experience as Dance*, 131. She also cites Forti, who argues Halprin was part of the San Francisco beat movement to which the Zen Master Suzuki Roshi was important. In 1964, Halprin became deeply involved with a psychoanalyst through whom she became profoundly influenced by Zen ideas. Ibid., 123.

57. *Moving Lessons*, 157.

58. Novack, *Sharing the Dance*, 183.

59. Halprin believed that she was denied access to modern dance because, despite showing great promise as a modern dancer training with Doris Humphrey, she was rejected from Bennington at a time when American universities were capping the number of Jewish students they would accept. Ross, *Experience as Dance*, 23.

60. Janice Ross recounts that when the dominant modern dance aesthetic impacted Wisconsin, where Halprin became a student after her rejection from Bennington, Halprin's resolve against the reigning aesthetic was strengthened. H'Doubler's methods provided Halprin with an alternative to the reigning modern dance avant-garde that she associated with her exclusion. When her student work was disparaged by a new faculty member, Halprin perceived the teacher as rejecting H'Doubler's approach. This was compounded by the fact that Bennington had recently become the first university to establish a dance program independent from physical education, with the founding logic that dance is high art as represented by the work of Graham, Humphrey, Charles Weidman, and Hanya Holm. Ibid., 108.

61. Halprin responded to the idea in Bauhaus that properties such as line, density, and space occur in the natural world. When Halprin had established her open-air studio in Northern California, she would have her students observe objects in the woods, such as plants or animals, and then ask them to use what they had seen in movement explorations without anticipating the outcome. Together, Halprin's use of the scientific and kinesthetic principles she learned from H'Doubler and the ideas about design that she gleaned from Bauhaus furnished her with the tools to develop a methodology for Movement Invention. Yet, the influence of Bauhaus also served to bolster Halprin's focusing of the dancer away from cultural specificity and toward the notion of nature as a benign source, so the various influences that she and her students may have had would be concealed within the notion of

exploring something outside of culture. Ibid., 65–66. Simone Forti recalls that, as Halprin's student, they would go into the forest around her outdoor deck and find shape and movement to emulate. Simone Forti, "Second Interview with Artist."

62. Mary Starks Whitehouse, "C.G. Jung and Dance Therapy: Two Major Principles," in *Authentic Movement: Essays by Mary Starks Whitehouse, Janet Adler and Joan Chodorow*, ed. Patrizia Pallaro (London: Jessica Kingsley Publishers, 1999), 74.

63. Janet Adler and Joan Chodorow, "Mary Stark Whitehouse's Papers," in *Authentic Movement: Essays by Mary Starks Whitehouse, Janet Adler and Joan Chodorow*, ed. Patrizia Pallaro (London: Jessica Kingsley Publishers, 1999), 14.

64. Mary Starks Whitehouse has written a whole chapter called "The Tao of the Body." Her student connects the idea in Authentic Movement of "direct experience" to Zen. Mary Starks Whitehouse, "The Tao of the Body," in *Authentic Movement: Essays by Mary Starks Whitehouse, Janet Adler and Joan Chodorow*, ed. Patrizia Pallaro (London: Jessica Kingsley Publishers, 1999), 41–50. Janet Adler, "Body and Soul," in *Authentic Movement: Essays by Mary Starks Whitehouse, Janet Adler and Joan Chodorow*, ed. Patrizia Pallaro (London: Jessica Kingsley Publishers, 1999), 166.

65. Joan Chodorow, "To Move and Be Moved," in *Authentic Movement: Essays by Mary Starks Whitehouse, Janet Adler and Joan Chodorow*, ed. Patrizia Pallaro (London: Jessica Kingsley Publishers, 1999), 269–70.

66. Mary Starks Whitehouse, "Creative Expression in Physical Movement Is Language without Words," in *Authentic Movement: Essays by Mary Starks Whitehouse, Janet Adler and Joan Chodorow*, ed. Patrizia Pallaro (London: Jessica Kingsley Publishers, 1999), 34.

67. Mary Starks Whitehouse, "Physical Movement and Personality," in *Authentic Movement: Essays by Mary Starks Whitehouse, Janet Adler and Joan Chodorow*, ed. Patrizia Pallaro (London: Jessica Kingsley Publishers, 1999), 52.

68. For a full discussion of the way in which Dunham's contribution was configured as specific rather than universal, see Morris, *A Game for Dancers*. In addition, Ramsay Burt shows how Dunham's project was one that attempted to recuperate identity for African Americans through ethnographic research that demonstrated that Africanist aesthetics had survived the Middle Passage. Explicating a rich cultural history is, however, inextricable from such a project. Ramsay Burt, *Alien Bodies: Representations of Modernity, "Race," and Nation in Early Modern Dance* (London: Routledge, 1998), 169–72.

69. Susan Manning, *Modern Dance, Negro Dance: Race in Motion* (Minneapolis: University of Minnesota Press, 2004).

70. Importantly, not all Somatics techniques that developed later in the twentieth century were influenced by modern dance. Feldenkrais Method is an important example, as it was developed as an approach to postural hygiene in its own right.

71. Bainbridge Cohen, *Sensing, Feeling, and Action: The Experiential Anatomy of Body-Mind Centering*, 3rd ed. (Northampton, MA: Contact Editions, 2012), 7–8.

72. F. M. Alexander tells the story of his healing in the 1932 text *The Use of Self* as the way in which he discovered his technique. The narrative became central to the teaching of his technique. Alexander recounts that professionals failed to help him with a voice loss problem he suffered as an actor and that he developed his training regimen from experiments he conducted to overcome the loss. Through deductive reasoning in observation of his corporeal action, he discovered that he was using his body counter to its natural propensity.

The solution was reorienting both his bodily action and consciousness to the logic of skeletal structure, an idea that became enshrined in the teaching of the technique. The methodology of Alexander's discovery is commonly recounted in a way that emphasizes the coming together of bodily knowledge and deductive reasoning. The pioneer is said to have worked alone with a series of mirrors watching what happened to his posture while he was delivering the lines from a theatrical text. It was in this process that he observed the way that he was holding himself with a "debauched" posture and concluded that he must execute better comportment. However, after observing that it was not possible to consciously direct the posture he desired, Alexander reported that he developed the technique in which the unconscious tendencies of the body and conscious will of the mind were brought together. Gelb, *Body Learning*, 11.

73. See, for example, the film *The Thinking Body: The Legacy of Mabel Todd*, in which the biography of Todd's personal discovery of the work is used to introduce her training, as taught by three prominent proponents of Ideokinesis. The story goes that after befalling a serious accident, medical doctors predicted Todd would never walk again. Yet, while convalescing, she experimented with ways of moving that would not cause pain and began to develop a new approach to the body as well as healing herself from her injuries. Loraine Corfield, Louise Williams, Nancy Topf, André Bernard, and Sally Swift, *The Thinking Body: The Legacy of Mabel Todd* (Piermont, NY: Teachers' Video Workshop, 1999), DVD.

74. Alexander narrates that he set up a series of mirrors so that he could observe himself from all sides when he gave himself instructions. He claims to have discovered that voluntary action in the body based on the idea of how his posture should be arranged did not work. He would observe that his body became arranged in a way that did not fulfill the postural habit toward which he was aiming. This is how Alexander insists he discovered a different way of working with the brain and the body, which needed to be instituted instead of instructed. Gelb, *Body Learning*.

75. For example, Alexander teacher June Ekman reports that she tried Graham technique in the 1950s but could not get the contraction and disliked the authoritarian approach. She was drawn to techniques working with ease, which she linked to Wilhelm Reich's psychoanalytical concept that the body functions as an emotional armor, and letting go of tension releases psychological blocks. Cunningham technique had become an important alternative to Graham technique for New York dancers, yet Ekman was not trained in ballet, which she felt was a necessity in Cunningham training. Consequently, she studied with Alwin Nikolais, who, influenced by Hanya Holm, was teaching what Ekman calls a more fluid swaying movement. She also took class with Lulu Sweigard teaching Ideokinesis and with Charlotte Selver teaching sensory awareness in the lineage of a practitioner known as Elsa Gintler. Ekman, "Discussion with the Author."

76. Ekman's distaste for Graham's and Cunningham's technique was based on the idea that working with effort compounded repression of the emotions and was psychologically unhealthy. Ibid. Elaine Summers was encouraged by her Jungian analyst to attend classes by Carola Speads and Charlotte Selver. Summer and Arnold, "Interview with Elaine Summers."

77. Rolland and Van Eijden, "Alignment and Release," 117.

78. Both Summers and Klein were prevented from launching careers as modern dancers due to injury. Summers, "Interview with Elaine Summers," and Susan Klein, "Klein Technique

History," Klein School, last modified 2005, http://kleintechnique.com/kt_history.pdf. Skinner danced for both Graham and Cunningham. She sustained an injury during her career, which she narrates as being so bad that she was told she could never dance again but recovered using Alexander Technique. Bridget Iona Davis, "Releasing into Process: Joan Skinner and the Use of Imagery in Dance" (MA thesis, University of Illinois, 1971). Skinner claims that she was only able to return to dancing by virtue of Alexander Technique, the ideas from which she applied to the ballet barre. She also cites Todd's work as an important influence and claims to have discovered a whole new way of dancing and training through her experiments. Bridget Davis is careful to point out that before Skinner took up Alexander Technique, she was questioning the way dance training seemed to work against natural bodily functions like breathing. "Releasing into Process," 14–24. In a more recent interview with Bettina Neuhaus, Skinner credits her initial childhood questioning of dance technique to the influence of the Todd-based classes. "The Kinaesthetic Imagination: An Interview with Joan Skinner," *Contact Quarterly Unbound*, 2010, https://contactquarterly. com/cq/unbound/view/skinner#. Nevertheless, the similarity between Skinner's exploration of dancing prior to the development of her technique and Alexander's textual representation of his process of "discovery" is striking. Davis narrates that prior to taking Alexander classes, Skinner had set up mirrors in a hallway in which she would observe what was happening in her body when she tried out the things that she was learning in dance class. Davis, "Releasing into Process." Klein emphasizes that the struggle of recovery following her injury process was both intellectual and physical. Bartenieff is the only Somatics influence she references along with acupuncture and the movement therapy "Zero Balancing." Klein characterizes her technique as the interface between formal dance training and bodywork. Klein lists her influences in her undated paper "Introduction to Klein Technique," https://kleintechnique.com/kt_Intro.pdf.

79. Both Klein and Skinner actually argue that their techniques are applicable to nondancers. However, Klein contends that her technique is unique because it was developed by and for dancers. Susan Klein, "Klein Technique: Application," Klein School, last modified 2005, http://kleintechnique.com/kt_application.pdf. Klein's claim seems unjustified because Skinner was also a dancer who developed her work specifically for dancers, a story that is recounted by Bridget Davis in her master's thesis. Davis, "Releasing into Process."

80. Mary Fulkerson reports reading a review of work at Judson in the early 1960s given to her by her high school dance teacher. Then, when she was a graduate student at the University of Illinois, where Joan Skinner was teaching, she met Paxton, who was on tour with the Cunningham Dance Company. Mary Fulkerson, "(Pioneer of Anatomical Releasing and Key Figure in the Dissemination of Somatics) in Discussion with the Author," interview by Doran George, May 31, 2012. Marsha Paludan and John Rolland, who also developed Anatomical Releasing, were student colleagues of Fulkerson at Illinois, so they would have also met Paxton and have been in conversation with Fulkerson about the new aesthetics.

81. Topf was teaching Cunningham Technique at the University of Illinois, where she noticed Rolland wobbling his head during class. He explained he was sensing the balance of his head on his spine, which intrigued Topf, who became involved with Rolland, Paludan, and Fulkerson. Buckwalter, "The Anatomy of Center."

82. Todd's text analyzes the body in component parts, such as "The Vertebral Pattern," on page 78, and "The Pelvic and Femoral Muscles," on page 118. She then applies the information to posture and motion of the whole structure, such as "Weight Bearing and Distribution in the Upright Position," on page 159. Todd, *The Thinking Body.*

83. The relationship to Cunningham training of the dancers using Somatics was complex because many of them continued to take Cunningham classes during their development of new approaches. For example, Fulkerson took classes when she could at Cunningham's studio while she was teaching at Rochester College in the early 1970s. They initially associated his training with his artistic perspective. Fulkerson, "Discussion with the Author."

84. Fulkerson recalls making the decision to explore new ideas when she began teaching at Rochester College in 1971 and acknowledges that this meant her students were not being trained to enter existing dance companies. Ibid.

85. Davis, "Releasing into Process," 19.

86. Skinner was so determined to prove that there was a new way to train dancers that she was initially resistant to having Mary Fulkerson join her classes. She told Fulkerson that she had too much technique, and Skinner wanted to show that she could train dancers from scratch. Fulkerson, "Discussion with the Author."

87. In addition to the evidence of this approach in the instructional lineage inherited from H'Doubler, the dance educator articulates this intention in her text *The Dance and Its Place in Education.* Ross, *Moving Lessons,* 133.

88. My knowledge of hands-on work is based on twenty years of taking Somatics classes with teachers such as Eva Karczag, Martha Moore, and others. I have verified that my experiences reflect the way that hands-on was used in the 1970s. Eva Karczag, "Eva Karczag (Dancer, Choreographer, Teacher) in Discussion with the Author," interview by Doran George, August 23–28, 2012.

89. Cohen had encouraged Goren and the other students to offer private sessions to dancers. Goren worked with people such as Judy Padow, Eva Karczag, Mary Overlie, Valda Setterfield, and Cynthia Hedstrom, all of whom became key figures in the artistic movement that combined somatics practice and new approaches to choreography. Beth Goren, "(B.M.C. Teacher) in Discussion with the Author," interview by Doran George, May 28, 2012.

90. For example, in Alexander Technique, it is called nondoing touch, and in Ideokinesis, it is often called tactile aid.

91. An example of Skinner's partnergraphics is the tracing of energy lines, like a sphere going up the back of the head and down the front of the face, which is informed by Alexandrian directions. My knowledge of this work is informed by twenty years of taking Skinner classes with teachers such as Stephanie Skura in the 1990s at Arnhem, Gaby Agis in London between 1998 and 2004, Yvonne Meier in New York from 2004 until 2010, and Lionel Popkin at UCLA in 2010 and 2012.

92. John Rolland suggests that such choreography was part of Barbara Clark's and André Bernard's teaching, both of whom were formulating their own versions of Todd's work. But Rolland insists that their classes were nevertheless more static than classes that he, Paludan, Fulkerson, and Todd developed for dance from Todd's work, including training from Clark and Bernard. Rolland and Van Eijden, "Alignment and Release," 119.

93. Davis reports that Skinner developed that technique through conversation with the students with whom she first began experimenting. Skinner recalls having developed exercises based on students' questions about how they could correct themselves following Skinner's introduction of principles of alignment into Graham-based classes. Davis narrates successive periods of experimentation and exchange between Skinner and her students, through which the class structure developed. Students would inform Skinner when they could and could not sustain an image within a given exercise. For example, they expressed difficulty keeping the image of a string that attaches from their head to the heavens while executing preset movement combinations. Skinner consequently developed a class structure with students that allowed them to work for long periods with an image and rarely used set movement. The idea that the exercises and class structure were guided by natural kinetic and sensory imperatives that arise in the connection between the human body-mind and the cosmos became embedded in the technique. Davis, "Releasing into Process."

94. Cohen, *Sensing, Feeling, and Action*, 3.

95. Goren, "Discussion with the Author." Daniel Lepkoff, "(Choreographer, Teacher) Discussion with the Author," interview by Doran George, August 24, 2011.

96. Dancers used the kinetics of the form to practice Somatics and felt CI demonstrated the possibilities of Somatics. For example, Lisa Kraus, who went on to dance for Trisha Brown in the late 1970s, reports having found little use for Somatics before she began applying the skills to CI and other improvisational methods Kraus studied at Bennington, from 1971 to 1974, when Paxton was in residence. Having been trained in dance since an early age, Kraus retained an appetite for large and challenging movement and was less interested in Paxton's inner stillness work. However, Bennington faculty, like Judith Dunn, inspired her interest in improvisation, which she fulfilled through combining Somatics and CI. Kraus was compelled by the different model of virtuosity in CI; she was excited by the notion of going from upright to rolling on the ground and moving with unpredictability in 360 degrees. CI gave her a kinesthetic experience that she wanted to work with solo. She took classes that used the simple kinetic structures offered by John Rolland's images because this enabled her to expand the experience of CI beyond the duet. Lisa Kraus, "(Dancer, Choreographer, Teacher) in Discussion with the Author," interview by Doran George, August 1, 2011. John Rolland, *Inside Motion: An Ideokinetic Basis for Movement Education*, rev. ed. (Amsterdam: Rolland String Research Associates, 1987).

97. In her notes, Novack cites an interview between Paxton and Banes in which the choreographer defined his project as seeking a way to apply the chance procedure to movement generation. Novack, *Sharing the Dance*, 54.

98. Ibid., 206.

99. Ibid., 74.

100. Novack argues that anxiety about potential injury precipitated changes in CI, whereby highly skilled dancing replaced a general rawness. Ibid., 79. She cites Lepkoff commenting that in the early experiments, the Rochester contingent were less subject to the kind of injury that many of the other early participants experienced because they had the facility to fall softly. Ibid., 65. The principles necessary to avoid injury could be found in Somatics practice. Novack chronicles an important development in CI as when practitioners

develop sophisticated strategies for falling, which allowed them to extend their skill level by taking more risks. Ibid., 151.

101. Deborah Jowitt, "Fall, You Will Be Caught," *Contact Quarterly* 3, no. 1 (Fall 1977): 28.

102. Paxton suggests that embodying concepts from physics through sensation is "'reality' as transcribed by subjective experience." Email correspondence with artist, September 20, 2011 (quotation marks from original).

103. Paxton, email correspondence with the artist (quotation marks from original).

104. Concerning the indirect influence of Somatics, Paxton, who is often credited as the inventor of CI, had little involvement directly in Somatics work. Yet, during the 1960s and early 1970s, he participated in artistic projects initiated by Brown and Forti, who brought the influence of Halprin, such as in the "Rule Games." Simone Forti, "First Discussion (Artist, Avant-Garde Luminary, and Teacher) with the Author," interview by Doran George, May 27, 2012.

105. Lionel Popkin recalls that the idea that humans are still in the process of evolving into upright posture was central to Klein's rhetoric. "Discussion with the Author."

106. Skinner has endorsed Bridget Davis's thesis that Skinner Releasing Technique intentionally works with the neuromuscular systems of alignment, balance, and mechanics of motion that Ideokinesis has identified as beyond conscious control. Davis's thesis has long been available on the Skinner Releasing website, which demonstrates that Skinner accepts the ideas. Davis, "Releasing into Process."

107. Bainbridge Cohen cites her work with spinal cord injury patients in whom feeling and motion were restored below the injury by her work with the organs. She argues that stimulating the viscera restores motor nerves because survival patterns, which manifest in organic functioning, are controlled by the autonomic nervous system that underlies the somatics nervous system. Bainbridge Cohen, *Sensing, Feeling, and Action*, 29.

108. For example, Bainbridge Cohen trained as an occupational therapist. Ibid. Susan Klein trained as an acupuncturist and in a technique called "Zero Balancing." Klein, "Klein Technique History." And practitioners who trained in Alexander Technique inherited the Alexander Lesson, which was designed as a one-on-one session. Gelb, *Body Learning*, 144.

109. David Held, *Models of Democracy*, 2nd ed. (Cambridge: Polity Press, 1998), 130–31.

110. Novack, *Sharing the Dance*.

111. This approach was particularly important in the various approaches fomented by Todd's work as well as in BMC and Authentic Movement.

112. Harraway has used the term in various publications. One source is "Modest_Witness@ Second_Millenium," in *Donna Haraway Reader*, (New York: Routledge, 2004), 223–50.

113. In Alexander's terms, CRP is thought to allow inhibition of the Startle Pattern so that a baseline can be established from which to recalibrate reasoning and volition. In Todd's work, the language used is different, but the idea is very similar.

114. Bridget Davis includes a description of an Alexander lesson in her thesis on Skinner Releasing. In it, students of Alexander Technique are encouraged to focus on the prompt or metaphor being given, since "sensation" is thought to be unreliable because kinesthesia is debauched. Davis, "Releasing into Process," 74–76.

115. June Ekman recalls that her first experience of Alexander Technique in the 1960s was one of not knowing how she had gotten up to standing after the massage/physical therapy work with the tactile support of an Alexander teacher. Ekman, "Discussion with the

Author." Similarly, David Hurwith reports that BMC teacher Beth Goren used her hands to elicit movement in his body that took him from lying to standing with no effort whatsoever in a way that eluded his consciousness of how the transition took place. David Hurwith, "(Dancer) in Discussion with the Author," interview by Doran George, May 6, 2012.

116. Gottschild, *Digging the Africanist Presence*, chapter 3.

117. My articulation of the way in which dancers constructed practices as non-Western and "Other" to their native culture is indebted to Edward Said's framework in *Orientalism*.

118. Paxton believed that by observing their reflexes calmly, dancers would cultivate experience that they could employ when they were in challenging and unfamiliar physical configurations. Paxton introduced the stand as a preparatory exercise for CI in the belief that the dancer would become "entrained" with the reflexes and therefore more able to meet physical disorientation without panic. Other exercises Paxton employed included inducing disorientation by asking students to move their heads into all the spaces around them gradually increasing the speed, practicing rolling with the eyes open, and remaining cognizant of the apparently turning room. Paxton, email correspondence with artist.

119. The first recorded performance of the stand is Paxton's 1972 *Mercury* at Oberlin College, often credited as the beginning of CI. Novack, *Sharing the Dance*, 61. While standing relatively still on two feet for a prolonged period, often with eyes closed, the practitioner inhibits the tendency to tense up against involuntary movement. Paxton suggests the exercise allows dancers to sense subtle shifts happening throughout their bodily structure and thereby develop "a persistent, delicate, overall awareness of the reflexes which balance the body." Paxton, email correspondence with artist.

120. Beth Goren remembers that she and many of the dancers who were practicing BMC were also taking classes with Klein in the 1970s. Goren, "Discussion with the Author."

121. Throughout the 1970s, Trisha Brown developed choreography informed by her work with Elaine Summers to reduce tension in her body. Her choreography demanded a conscious and complex understanding of the dancing body. Summers and Arnold, *Interview with Elaine Summers*. Then in 1981, as Philip Bother argues, a turning point in Brown's career occurred when Harvey Lichtenstein invited her to present *Glacial Decoy* at the Brooklyn Academy of Music, alongside Lucinda Childs, whose dancers were also training in Somatics, and Laura Dean. This was Brown's first large concert hall performance in the United States. Philip Bither, "From Falling and Its Opposite, and All the In-Betweens," Walker Arts Center, 2013, http://www.walkerart.org/magazine/2013/philip-bither-trisha-brown.

122. Kraus comments that when she first started dancing for Trisha Brown, she was swimming in a swamp of Somatics, and Brown's structures gave her a form through which to articulate the skills she had developed. Kraus, "Discussion with the Author."

123. In the late 1970s, Kraus used anatomical prompts when she began teaching LOCUS in and beyond New York. Diane Madden, "(Dancer and Teacher, and Rehearsal Director with Trisha Brown Dance Company) in Discussion with Artist," interview by Doran George, May 25, 2012.

124. Ibid.

125. Many teachers, as I have mentioned before, used CRP from Alexander and Ideokinesis. Diane Madden, Jeremy Nelson, Neil Greenberg, and others began using the slow rolldown over the legs that is characteristic of Klein Technique. Ibid.

126. For example, Diane Madden, who danced alongside Karczag in Brown's company, reports that she transposed ideas from Alexander Technique to formal class, such as a set of prompts called "directions." Other Brown dancers, such as Iréne Hultman, Vicky Shick, and later Shelly Senter, used similar strategies, as did Petronio dancers, such as Jeremy Nelson. Madden, "Discussion with Artist."

127. Vicky Shick, email correspondence, February 9, 2014.

128. These descriptions are based on correspondence with Shick. Ibid.

129. Madden recalls that Brown provided the movement or gave directions on how to make the movement, but it was up to the dancer to find a way of executing the dance. Madden, "Discussion with Artist."

130. For example, dancers in Lucinda Child's and Stephen Petronio's companies both used Alexander and/or Klein at different times.

131. Karczag joined Trisha Brown's company in the late 1970s, bringing with her experience of studying Alexander Technique as well as Tai Chi in the United Kingdom. She became a strong proponent of its value for the performance of Brown's choreography, which was convincing for company members and Brown herself. Elizabeth Garren, whom Karczag replaced in the company, had already been working with Alexander Technique. Karczag, "Discussion with the Author."

132. Karczag had substantial experience in both Graham technique and classical ballet, which she had trained in and performed, for example, with the London Festival Ballet, for which she had moved from Australia to England in the early 1970s. Ibid.

133. Ibid.

134. Deborah Jowitt, "By Deborah Jowitt (Eva Karczag)," *Village Voice*, March 8, 1994.

135. Along with Karczag, Madden, as well as Iréne Hultman, Shelley Senter, and many other company members, took up Alexander Technique, many as students of June Ekman. Ekman, "Discussion with the Author."

136. Madden, "Discussion with the Artist."

137. Voluntary activity is thought to recapitulate habitual postural schema because the sensory feedback mechanism, by which action is executed, has been incorrectly habituated. It is argued that knowledge of executing an action is drawn from sensation based on previous experience that has invariably been conditioned by the Startle Pattern in a goal-oriented culture. See, for example, descriptions of unreliable sensory appreciation and "inhibition." Gelb, *Body Learning*, 52–67.

138. Madden, "Discussion with the Artist."

139. Stephen Petronio introduced Madden to Klein's work when she began having back problems in the early 1980s, when she began dancing for Brown full time. Madden was already doing Alexander Technique at the time. Ibid.

140. Ibid.

141. For example, in workshops that Eva Karczag taught, it was common for there to be a time in the class when dancers who had trained in classical or modern techniques would talk about the liberation they were achieving through Somatics.

142. For example, Ekman taught Iréne Hultman, Diane Madden, Shelley Senter, Eva Karczag, and Lionel Popkin, all of whom danced with Trisha Brown and Jeremy Nelson, who danced for Stephen Petronio. Ekman, "Discussion with the Author."

143. Charlip, with whom Ekman had danced, started Alexander training together with Ekman in 1977. Eckman met Karczag through Trisha Brown and also because Elizabeth Garren, whose place Eva took in the company, was in the same training as Eckman. Ibid.

144. Ekman and her colleagues went to some trouble to bring Barstow to teach for a New York dance community interested in Somatics. Barstow was seen as something of a renegade by the Alexander community, and Ekman was able to gather support to bring her to New York because of the interest in the dance community. Ibid. Karczag suggests that people taught Alexander very differently from each other. Karczag herself brought to her teaching of Alexander Technique her work with Fulkerson and a Tai Chi master, named Gerder Gedders. She remarks that the teachers she was drawn to in the United States, such as Ekman and Barstow, exhibited a more flowing approach to the technique than many Alexander teachers. She also proposed that the technique is taught in a more rigid way in the United Kingdom than the United States. Karczag, "Discussion with the Author."

145. This is a description that Ishmael Houston-Jones gave of the event. "(Choreographer and Artist) in Discussion with the Author," interview by Doran George, June 6, 2012.

146. Peter Rose spent a summer in Poland working with Jerzy Grotowski, who had abandoned the idea of performance because he found what was happening in the rehearsal process more compelling. Based on his experience of Grotowski's ideas, Rose inaugurated the weekly meeting place for dancers at the recently established performance and rehearsal space PS 122 in New York's East Village. Stephanie Skura, "(Choreographer and Teacher) in Discussion with the Author," interview by Doran George, May 13, 2013.

147. The improvisational technique of dancing was integrated with text and other practices in several experimental events that were neither performance nor class. "Open Presentation" was started by Skura and Russell, in which artists would try an idea; at "Night Reading," artists shared text from their journals, sometimes more than one reading simultaneously; and at "Avantgardarama," artists would try out ideas. Ibid.

148. At "Avantgardarama," Houston-Jones danced on Second Avenue asking the audience to watch him from the windows of PS 122. Skura remarks how intense it was to see him moving vigorously while the lights of cars whizzed by. She performed the making of an omelette in PS 122's kitchen, inviting the audience to sample her cooking as part of the performance. Ibid.

149. Meier heard about the technique from dancer and writer Tim Miller, who was Meier's roommate in New York and had worked with Skinner in Seattle, where she based after leaving Illinois. Meier attended a regular summer workshop that Skinner had begun to teach and immediately began teaching Skinner Releasing when she returned to New York. Ibid.

150. Working with the same image, dancers might be lying completely still on the floor or dancing wildly. The idea was to listen to the body and allow it to follow the energy on a particular day rather than trying to emulate a particular idea of how the image works. Davis, "Releasing into Process," 59.

151. Whitehouse reports she rediscovered the value of the lost legacy of modern dance in Jungian psychoanalysis. She realized the body is the location of the unconscious and the proper vehicle for expression of the psyche, which is why dance has such creative potential. Jungian psychoanalysis configures Western culture as impeding the authentic self. Whitehouse suggests that objective knowledge as well as stereotyped notions of right and wrong must be disbanded as students listen to their psyche with no preconceived idea of where the work will take them. Frieda Sherman, "Conversation with Mary Whitehouse," in *Authentic Movement: Essays by Mary Starks Whitehouse, Janet Adler and Joan Chodorow*, ed. Patrizia Pallaro (London: Jessica Kingsley Publishers, 1999), 29–32.
152. The witness–mover dyad is based on the psychoanalytic process. Whitehouse's student Janet Adler argues that movers internalize the witness and learn to differentiate between authentic bodily responses and projecting and fulfilling an image by observing themselves moving. Janet Adler, "Who Is the Witness? A Description of Authentic Movement," in *Authentic Movement: Essays by Mary Starks Whitehouse, Janet Adler and Joan Chodorow*, ed. Patrizia Pallaro (London: Jessica Kingsley Publishers, 1999), 153–55.
153. Codified language exists for this part of the process, which is designed to abate judgment in either negative or positive terms. Judgment is thought to obstruct the process of reaching for the authentic self because it inhibits the free flow of the psyche. (Author's personal reflections from classes)
154. Whitehouse argues that movers have to let go of preconceptions they have about what looks attractive or how they think they should move. Frieda Sherman, "Conversation with Mary Whitehouse," in *Authentic Movement: Essays by Mary Starks Whitehouse, Janet Adler and Joan Chodorow*, ed. Patrizia Pallaro (London: Jessica Kingsley Publishers, 1999), 30.

   She suggests that staying tuned to "honest bodily" reaction is a process that entails the practitioner learning to identify when they "arrange" movement. She asserts that the unconscious source of the dance is evidenced by its initiation from an impulse within the body that is distinct from conscious decision making. Mary Starks Whitehouse, "Physical Movement and Personality," in *Authentic Movement: Essays by Mary Starks Whitehouse, Janet Adler and Joan Chodorow*, ed. Patrizia Pallaro (London: Jessica Kingsley Publishers, 1999), 51–57.
155. Jennifer Miller, "(Choreographer, Dancer, S.U.N.Y. Purchase Faculty) in Discussion with Artist," interview by Doran George, August 18, 2011.
156. Ishmael Houston-Jones commented that when he saw a video of himself in a ballet class in the mid-1970s, he was repelled by the mannered look of his dancing and ceased from training in the technique. Houston-Jones, "Discussion with the Author." Jennifer Monson found solace in Somatics coming from a university dance program where she was on parole because the ballet-based aesthetic of the faculty deemed her overweight. "(Choreographer, Dancer, Teacher) in Discussion with the Author," interview by Doran George, July 23–27, 2011. In the same time period, Stephanie Skura experienced problems imposed by the balletic aesthetic at New York University's Tisch dance program, where she was encouraged as a choreographer but felt undervalued as a dancer because her feet lacked a proper arch. "Discussion with the Author."
157. Fulkerson recalls that during the early experiments, Skinner's images were simpler and less poetic. "Discussion with the Author."

158. Skinner's beliefs about poetry and the function of the image are expressed in the article "The Depth of Openness: A Study of Deep Image Poetry." The author, George Gleason, argues poetic images drawn from the collective unconscious transfer energy to the reader, which is then transformed back into kinesthetic form. Joan Skinner, *Teacher Training Reader* (Seattle Skinner Releasing Teacher Certification Program, undated), 25.

159. Bainbridge Cohen explicitly references Todd as an influence in *Sensing, Feeling and Action*, 158.

160. Ibid., 30.

161. The importance of chi is evident in the role that the "meridian stretches" came to play for teachers such as Eva Karczag, Lisa Kraus, and Iréne Hultman. The training provided them with a way of connecting a simple stretch series with the movement energy along the meridian lines in the body, which were represented as energy circuits in traditional Chinese medicine. For Karczag, the meridian stretches also connected with her use of Tai Chi. Ilchi Lee, *Meridian Exercise for Self-Healing*, Dahnhak, the Way to Perfect Health Series, 2 vols. (Las Vegas: Healing Society, 2003). Meanwhile, Susan Klein, Bonnie Bainbridge Cohen, and many other teachers refer to the chakras in their work.

162. My knowledge of Karczag's work is gleaned from taking class with her at the European Dance Development Center, in Arnhem, Holland, between 1992 and 1996, and also participating in workshops she taught in London, in 2000, at Moving East Studio, and New York, in 2008, at the Trisha Brown Dance Studio, and in 2010, through Movement Research. She has also verified my analysis in interview and via email.

163. Susan Leigh Foster points out that corporate, as opposed to state, funding, which became the dominant source of patronage for the arts as the twentieth century progressed, diminishes experimentation in a variety of ways. *Dances That Describe Themselves: The Improvised Choreography of Richard Bull* (Middletown, CT: Wesleyan University Press, 2002), 131–39.

164. McKenzie cites "managing diversity" as a performance model that became popular toward the end of the twentieth century and saw inclusion of cultural and social variety as contributing to the performance capability of organizations. *Perform or Else*, 68.

165. Melanie Bales articulates the shift in training, although she does not link it to changes in the conception of self to political and economic ideas. Melanie Bales, "A Dancing Dialectic," in *The Body Eclectic: Evolving Practices in Dance Training*, ed. Melanie Bales and Rebecca Nettl-Fiol (Urbana: University of Illinois Press, 2008), 16–17.

166. For example, Karczag left Brown's company when it began securing gigs in large spaces because she felt that framing of the work within the conventional separation of choreographer and dancer replaced evidence of her creative contribution when the intimacy between the performer and audience was lost. She was not prepared to sacrifice her participation in direct democracy. Karczag, "Discussion with the Author."

167. For example, Lionel Popkin felt that Klein's ideas were knitted into Brown's choreography. He felt that learning to be grounded through bony connection contributed to his ability to execute vocabulary that was created by dancers like Madden and Brown herself, who were influenced by Klein training. Popkin, "Discussion with the Author."

168. Siobhan Davis undertook a similar initiative in London in 2006.

169. It is notable in Movement Research that teachers of daily technique class were generally dancers with companies, and those teaching workshops were more likely to be independent artists not working on concert stages with conventional approaches to composition. Movement Research, *Movement Research Performance Journal* (New York: Movement Research, 1990). Similarly, in London, teachers giving daily technique class through Independent Dance, in the 1990s, were generally those dancing for Siobhan Davis or Rosemary Butcher, such as Gill Clarke, or those with small companies making conventional work informed by Somatics, such as Fin Walker and Gregory Nash.

170. For example, while he was dancing for Terry Creach and auditioning and apprenticing for Trisha Brown, Lionel Popkin recalls he used Klein Technique to "clean out" his body. When he was dancing for Brown, he didn't want to take a class in which he was learning material; he wanted to warm up in a way that would last for six hours. He suggests that Klein's work warmed up his bones. Popkin, "Discussion with the Author."

171. This is evident, for example, in the fact that, alongside the regular classes at Brown's studio, special workshops were taught by educators who focused on movement principles, such as Susan Klein and Eva Karczag. The positioning of these workshops, as marginal to the regular daily class, frame them as complementary to the more conventional skills associated with "technique class." (I have attended such workshops and followed them on Brown's studio program over the last twelve years.)

172. Popkin recounts that the different roles created by dancers such as Karczag and Randy Warshaw made very different demands on the dancers. He felt that he brought very different skills to the table than company members with extensive classical training, and the uniqueness of each dancer was put to use in the assigning of roles in repertory. Popkin, "Discussion with the Author."

173. Popkin recalls that when he was in Brown's company, from 2000 to 2003, the dancers pursued their own training preferences, some of which were Somatics based and others that were ballet and yoga. Popkin, "Discussion with the Author."

174. Netl-Fiol and Vanier, *Dance and the Alexander Technique: Exploring the Missing Link*, xiii.

175. Skinner officially began her teacher training in 1991, although Stephanie Skura recalls that some people went through a training before then. Skura, Facebook message to the author, November 29, 2013. Klein's training began at least as early as 1994, when Neil Greenberg joined. Greenberg, email correspondence, September 24, 2013.

176. Goren, "Discussion with the Author."

177. The emphasis upon process is compounded by the inclusion of exchanges by letters Bainbridge Cohen has had with students. Bainbridge Cohen, *Sensing, Feeling, and Action*.

178. Mary Starks Whitehouse, "Reflections on a Metamorphosis," in *Authentic Movement: Essays by Mary Starks Whitehouse, Janet Adler and Joan Chodorow*, ed. Patrizia Pallaro (London: Jessica Kingsley Publishers, 1999), 58–62.

179. For example, in 1999, shortly after Greenberg was certified, his teaching privileges were revoked because he disagreed with Klein and Mahler. Greenberg, email correspondence. More recently, Skura has also felt the need to establish her own approach independently from Skinner. Skura, "Discussion with the Author." These shifts in the regimens parallel the resentment that Novack identified in 1980s CI, when dancers broke with antihierarchical ethics by establishing reputations as teachers, although the CI community continually refused to establish teacher certification. Novack, *Sharing the Dance*, 220–21.

180. Exchanges in *Movement Research Performance Journal*, between Karczag and Klein, reflect disagreement over the authority of the principles associated with the Alexander and Klein Techniques, respectively. In a workshop that I took in London in 2000, Klein gave participants the articles as reading material (Workshop at Greenwich Dance Agency, London, September 2000).

181. I heard about this in late 1990s London from Fin Walker, a British choreographer and dancer who was a prominent figure in the development of Somatics. The discussion in London happened at a time when significant numbers of British dancers were being exposed to Klein Technique for the first time. Gill Clarke, another British dancer and choreographer, who was a prominent figure in the development of Somatics, also openly discussed the merits and pitfalls of Klein compared with Alexander Technique.

182. Jeremy Nelson, who is now teaching at a conservatory in Denmark, began teaching at P.A.R.T.S. in the 1990s, along with other New York dancers. Jeremy Nelson, email correspondence, February 9, 2014. Gill Clarke who danced for Siobhan Davis, began teaching her Alexander-influenced approach at Trinity Laban in the same decade. I know this information from personal contact with all the artists mentioned over at least a fifteen-year period.

183. For example, Monson, Houston-Jones, Sarah Skaggs, Neil Greenberg, Tere O'Conner, and Kirstie Simson began working as adjuncts, many of them eventually occupying tenured positions.

184. Exercises in the Klein studio are slow, careful, sustained, minimal actions designed to isolate and move specific body parts and nurture weighted connection through the bones. A "connected" body never loses its sense of weight that transfers into the floor and up through the skeleton. Klein argues that when weighted connection is sustained in challenging choreography, dancers have greater fullness, ease, efficiency, and, in fact, beauty of motion. Susan Klein, "Dancing from the Spirit," *Movement Research Performance Journal* 13 (Fall 1996): 20.

185. In Klein Technique, energy is accessed by connecting differentiated tissues of the body, which is established as weight transfers effectively through the pelvis into the legs. A "knowing state" emerges through proper connection to the earth, which parallels Alexander's and Todd's insistence that consciousness is coeval with upright posture. Like Skinner, Klein places importance of connection not only within the body and between the body and the earth but also between people and, in fact, between everything in the universe. And in a similar way to BMC, the various component parts of the body are given psychological value. Klein Technique is, therefore, presented as a process in which spiritual work of the highest order is done, exhibiting a kind of morality that is exhibited throughout most of the Somatics practices. Klein, "Dancing from the Spirit."

186. Like Klein, Bainbridge Cohen references the Laban/Bartenieff lineage as an influence on her work, which may explain some of the similarities such as the use of the term "knowing" and her particular idea about the mind being distinct from the body, even while she aims to achieve their unity through restoring the "natural" relationship between them. Bainbridge Cohen, *Sensing, Feeling, and Action*, 1–4.

187. The goal of a "knowing state" is achieved through connection among all tissue levels to the deepest, which is manifest in the bone. Techniques, or styles, that focus on superficial muscle impede an individual's development on every level. Somatics' critique of

force associated with Graham technique was based in the idea that it used only superficial muscle.

188. In the 1990s, Bebe Miller taught regularly at Movement Research, David Rousseve and his dancers trained at the Klein studio, and David Zambrano developed Flying Low technique. Julie Tolentino, "(Dancer and Artist) in Discussion with the Author," interview by Doran George, April 7, 2014.

189. Butoh artists Eiko and Koma taught regularly through Movement Research, and the program also featured the Urban Bush Women and African dance taught by Paul Kengmo. But the majority of classes were Somatics-based training. Movement Research, *Movement Research Performance Journal*.

190. Karczag remembers that teaching the 1980s work by Brown, *Set and Reset*, in which she was part of the original cast, she focused on aptitudes that had been important to her as a dancer. Vicky Shick, another original cast member, actually came to teach the set movement because it was not Karczag's strength. Eva Karczag, email correspondence, May 27, 2014.

191. The way in which Orientalism and primitivism work together in the construction of an invisible category of the natural body deserves further investigation. In her critique of the term "postmodern," Ananja Chatterjea articulates the concept "women of color," which draws useful alliances between bodies that are subject primarily to Orientalism and those that have suffered a history of primitivist projection. Ananya Chatterjea, *Butting Out: Reading Resistive Choreographies through Works by Jawole Willa Jo Zollar and Chandralekha* (Middletown, CT: Wesleyan University Press, 2004). Brenda Dixon Gottschild provides a useful counterpoint to Chatterjea because she insists that Africanisms have been "disappeared" in American culture, unlike the contribution made by Asian cultures. Chatterjea's *Butting Out* may in some way be a rejoinder to Gottschild because in it, the author points out the ways in which women of color, including Asian bodies, are made to signify history and culture in the context of the postmodern from which they are consequently excluded. The way that Orientalism and primitivism function together in Somatics suggests that Gottschild's and Chatterjea's frameworks may speak to different sides of a common issue: bodies marked as having African decent are configured as the raw humanity to which bodies configured as Eastern have a historical connection through theè ancient cultures. But, because of the signifying functions accorded to nonwhite bodies, they are excluded from bringing raw and ancient knowledge together in the production of a sophisticated modern present.

Chapter 2

1. German modern dance contributed to Somatics in all the transnational hubs. The reduction of tension in Somatics is indebted to an instructional lineage of German teachers. Some midcentury New York dancers exploring the reduction of tension also turned to Hanya Holm's work, which they felt was more flowing and easier on the body compared with Graham technique. Yet, postwar acknowledgment of German influence would have been problematic, despite exiled modern teachers bringing information to all the transnational hubs. British late twentieth-century choreographers who contributed to the uptake

of Somatics experimented with bodily tension through Laban's work before they were exposed to American ideas. Laban disseminated his ideas in the United Kingdom while he was in exile, which had widespread influence through the high school system. Karczag and Anne Thompson also report that classes they took as children taught by German moderns influenced their interest in Somatics in adult life. Laban's work was also important in the development of artists such as Rosemary Butcher, Sue Maclennan, and Janet Smith, all of whom went on to be crucial in the development of dance in Britain that became associated with Somatics. All the artists refer to Laban's ideas that they were exposed to at Dartington in the late 1960s, which were not based on a predetermined vocabulary and worked with the tone of the body in a way that ultimately became associated with Somatics. Yet, in postwar modern dance, German influence was underplayed, if not erased, because of hostility following the global conflict. Valerie Preston-Dunlop points out in her film, *The American Invasion, 1962–1972*, that modern dance struggled to emerge in postwar Britain precisely because of its association with Germany. All the transnational hubs were allies against Germany in World War II, so it is likely they felt equal hostility toward German cultural forms. Valerie Preston-Dunlop and Luis España, *The American Invasion, 1962–1972* (Friends of the Laban Centre, 2005), DVD, 108 min.

2. The postwar text *The Vital Center* exemplifies such ideas. Authored by Arthur Schlesinger, political historian and adviser to Franklin D. Roosevelt and the Kennedy brothers, among other prominent politicians, it exemplifies the centrality of New York City. My reference to Schlesinger builds on Serge Guilbaut's scholarship in *How New York Stole the Idea of Modern Art: Abstract Expressionism, Freedom, and the Cold War*. He maintains that the global success of New York visual art depended on Schlesinger's ideas. America, Guilbaut asserts, internationally promoted its painters to showcase the fruits of creative freedom in line with Schlesinger's insistence that mature societies tolerate cultural dissidence. Guilbaut, *How New York Stole the Idea of Modern Art*. Boosters of modern painting and the government verified American liberalism by promoting artists that were vilified by the domestic establishment. Ibid., 184.

3. The way that Somatics traveled to the three non-American countries can be traced to just a few people. In 1972, the American artist and educator Mary Fulkerson introduced Somatics, which she had begun developing in New England, to the United Kingdom. She became a linchpin for a first wave of dissemination that had begun in Europe. American-trained Dutch dancer Pauline De Groot connected with Fulkerson and other Americans to support Somatics education in the Netherlands, following her return there in 1969. In 1976, Nanette Hassall, Russell Dumas, and Eva Karczag introduced Somatics to their Australian homeland.

4. The do-it-yourself approach to dissemination also depended on government expansionism because Somatics rode on the coattails of American modern dance. As Naima Prevots points out in her study of the use of modern dance as a form of cultural diplomacy, the state began funding international tours of Martha Graham's and José Limón's companies in the 1950s. Prevots, *Dance for Export*. They intended to export liberalism and change perceptions of America as unsophisticated, insular, and only interested in profit. Britain and Holland, where modern dance had not been consistently sustained, rapidly took up the American tradition. Graham protégés helped establish training institutions in the late 1960s. Within just a few years, Somatics proponents used America's significance as

the origin of modern dance with the idea that the regimens originated in New York as the newest development.

5. Cunningham independently funded his first international tour in 1964 after a decade's rejection by the government panel for funding, which was populated by the dance-establishment. Prevots, *Dance for Export*, 53–58. He had also lacked support from the domestic press and concert houses. Lewis Lloyd, email correspondence. He had been deemed as failing the modernist universality of staging emotion, myth, and symbol. Prevots, *Dance for Export*, 55–56. Yet, after his international success, the modern-oriented establishment was forced to accept Cunningham's artistic credibility by virtue of his avant-garde dissidence, and the constitution of universality was fundamentally challenged.

6. Key figures in the transnational development of Somatics witnessed the role of "internationalism" in Cunningham's struggle with and eventual embrace by the American dance establishment.

7. Guilbaut articulates that for both New York and Parisian postwar commentators on literature, architecture, and painting, the expression of a uniquely national perspective that spoke to international rather than domestic concerns was crucial to the establishment of high culture. Guilbaut, *How New York Stole*, 43–44.

8. Critique became intertwined with elitism for the midcentury avant-garde when choreographers who rejected 1950s institutionalized modernism also recharacterized the masses in their refusal to pander to large audiences. Leftist dancers of the 1930s had believed in the revolutionary potential of the proletariat, as exemplified in the communicative transparency of their socialist-realist choreography. Yet, as leftist dance collapsed, accessibility became the purview of modern dance, which had previously only reached small audiences of devotees. Responding to the imposition of modern dance universality and the attendant idea of communicability, the avant-garde recharacterized the masses as a reactionary middle-class force against which dissidence was defined. For example, Rebekah Kowal argues that Cunningham rejected mass conformity in Cold War containment culture. Kowal, *How to Do Things with Dance*. Dissidence was consolidated as critique for the American Left during the Cold War, most vividly in the devastation reeked by McCarthy. In a related move, a concerted effort at concert dance opacity, such as Cunningham's, resisted establishment dictates exemplified in the narrative clarity of Graham. Scholars such as Kowal have argued that despite the racial biases by which the midcentury avant-garde has been enshrined, and its critique deemed successful, choreographers still launched gender and queer critique even when such references were averted. Ibid.

9. Thinly veiled elitism can be read into the projects of early 1960s Greenwich Village artists who, Sally Banes argues, inverted the values of the suburban masses in what she calls "heterotopias." Sally Banes, *Greenwich Village 1963: Avant-Garde Performance and the Effervescent Body* (Durham, NC: Duke University Press, 1993), 13.

10. Mary Fulkerson, for example, narrates that her development was influenced by seeing a news clipping about Judson in the 1960s, and although she was never permanently based in New York, she became associated with many of the artists whose early development happened in Greenwich Village in the early 1960s. Fulkerson, "Discussion with the Author."

11. A key text was Sally Banes's *Terpsichore in Sneakers: Post-Modern Dance* (Boston: Houghton Mifflin, 1980), which functioned like a glossary of Judson artists and their approaches.

12. De Groot, "Discussion with the Author."

13. Paxton, Forti, and Nelson had relocated to New England in the 1970s, while Fulkerson, among others, had never based herself in New York. Their location in New England was either collapsed into New York or understood as respite from the metropolis, and therefore related to the centrality of New York City. At the same time, the background in Somatics of artists, such as the British choreographer Rosemary Butcher, disappeared into the significance of New York once they had visited the city. Before she encountered American Somatics, Butcher trained in Laban's work along with other artists who became significant in the development of the work in Britain.

14. A respected national newspaper reviewing *Glacial Decoy* charged that "anyone moderately active could have mastered the little runs, jumps, bursts of energy." Clare Hayes, "Review of Glacial Decoy," *New Dance Magazine* 12 (1979): 26. Writing in *New Dance Magazine*, Clare Hayes cites this quote from Mary Clarke writing for *The Guardian* national newspaper. Ibid. By 1984, the mainstream publication *The Dancing Times*, known for its heavily ballet-focused aesthetic, included a glowing review of Brown's "Set and Reset," by Alistair McCauley, "Umbrelldom," *Dancing Times*, January 1984, 302.

15. Paxton taught at the X6 studio and Dartington festival (Claid, *Yes? No! Maybe . .* , 2006, 83) in the same year he programmed at London's premier dance festival Dance Umbrella. Jack Anderson, *Choreography Observed* (Iowa City: University of Iowa Press, 1987), 182.

16. Jeremy Nelson consistently taught for Movement Research and also taught in marginal contexts in London that sustained Somatics, such as the Greenwich Dance Agency and European Dance Development Center.

17. I am mentioning Pooh Kaye, which I did not do in chapter 1 on training, because she made her contribution through choreography rather than training. But she is significant because, as I detail in chapter 3, her style influenced East Village developments through dancers such as Monson, Meier, and David Zambrano, who developed the "Flying Low Technique," which exhibits elements of her choreographic approach. Kaye actually discovered Somatics training through her dancers, such as Meier, who introduced Skinner Releasing and began teaching warm-up. Pooh Kaye, "(Choreographer, Dancer, Filmmaker) in Discussion with the Author," interviewed by Doran George, August 15, 2011.

18. In a review of Houston-Jones's 1985 work *Them*, one writer suggested that the reworking of CI created violent images of homosexual encounters. Robert Sandla, "À La Recherche Des Tricks Perdue," *Movement Research Performance Journal* 38 (2011 [1986]): 19–20.

19. For example, in the early 1990s, improviser Kate Brown, who was my first improvisation teacher (1989), talked about feeling alienated in London because her aesthetic related to East Village dance, which she had connected with in New York in the 1980s. Furthermore, beginning in the 1990s, artists with small state grants independently curated performances and workshops by Houston-Jones, Monson, Meier, and others at Chisenhale Dance Space. At Chisenhale Dance Space, I participated in a workshop/performance with Houston-Jones, in 1999, curated by Gaby Agis, and I curated my own series with Jennifer Monson and Yvonne Meier in 2000. Houston-Jones and Monson recalled teaching earlier workshops during numerous interviews with me between 2008 and 2014.

20. The centrality of New York choreography is demonstrated in the late 1970s and early 1980s by the programming for London's Dance Umbrella festival. Despite being the largest global endeavor of its kind for contemporary work during that period, New York artists were

disproportionately represented at Dance Umbrella because the American city was perceived as the locus of the greatest industry and sophistication in the art form. Stephanie Jordan, *Striding Out: Aspects of Contemporary and New Dance in Britain* (London: Dance Books, 1992), 100.

21. The crucial roles of Halprin, on the West Coast, and Skinner, in Illinois, are just two examples of many.

22. Summers, Bainbridge Cohen, Clark, Topf, and Bernard all taught a burgeoning new generation of New York dancers in the 1970s, many of whom were also training in CI. Summers, Bainbridge Cohen, and Paxton all rapidly became known as Somatics pioneers throughout the transnational network, and Ideokinesis was seen as an important technique associated with Todd.

23. Skinner developed her Releasing Technique in Illinois and Seattle, and it only became well known when it was introduced to New York in the 1980s. Gaby Agis first brought the work to England after she encountered it in New York, and similarly, Skinner's approach was only taught in the Netherlands because of visiting artists from New York such as Skura and Meier. Gaby Agis, "(Choreographer, Dancer, Teacher) in Discussion with the Author," interview by Doran George, September 7, 2012.

24. Fulkerson and De Groot both developed Somatics pedagogies in the 1960s but were never recognized to the same degree within the transnational community because they focused on British and Dutch hubs, rather than New York City.

25. The link is exemplified in the way that 1970s Somatics practitioners understood the training to be crucial to Brown's choreography, which was recapitulated in the 1990s with Stephen Petronio's work. Brown's artistic approach was associated with Somatics because from the late 1970s onward dancers taught her choreography along with Somatics ideas. The look of Brown's dances also contrasted with classical and modern approaches in a way that seemed to exhibit Somatics aptitudes.

26. Brown did not give her dancers classes and rarely taught repertory outside of the company. Instead, she asked her dancers to fulfill that role. The use that Brown's dancers made of Somatics in their teaching of her work is not surprising because the artists first developed her vocabulary during intensive study of Summers' Kinetic Awareness work, which she insisted her dancers also follow in the late 1970s. As discussed in chapter 1, these dancers, left to their own devices, in subsequent decades practiced and taught Alexander and Klein Technique, which became well known throughout the Somatics network. While continuing dance, company members such as Karczag, Irène Hultman, and Shelley Senter trained as Alexander teachers, and Diane Madden along with Stephen Petronio became devotees of Klein Technique, which they incorporated into their teaching.

27. Claid, *Yes? No! Maybe . . .*, 83, and Jordan, *Striding Out*, 93.

28. In Britain, in the late 1970s, the association between Contact Improvisation and Anatomical Releasing was so strong that dancers called the work "Contact Release." Mara De Wit, "New Dance Development at Dartington College of Arts U.K. 1971–1987" (PhD diss., Middlesex University, 2000).

29. De Groot reports that many of her students were not concerned with dance as a serious endeavor, which contributed to her isolation in the Netherlands and possibly influenced her commitment to working in an institutional modern dance program despite difficulties. De Groot, "Discussion with the Author." Both Miranda Tufnell and Karczag also recall that a significant proportion of their students in Britain and Australia, respectively,

were interested in the alternative healing scene as much as dance. De Wit, "New Dance Development at Dartington," 159; Karczag, "Discussion with the Author."

30. Workshops that Brown, Petronio, or their company members taught in association with the school cemented the idea that, above all the other Somatics approaches, Klein Technique was singularly directed to professionalism within contemporary dance.

31. Throughout the last forty years of the twentieth century, ballet continued to be acceptable training for New York dancers using Somatics. Not all dancers attended classical training, but the approach was not taboo for dancers working with Somatics in dominant New York discourse, which was distinct from the Netherlands, for example.

32. Although releasing approaches marked a departure from the modern dance vocabularies, Klein claimed her approach supported dancers' execution of any "style," including Graham, Cunningham, and Limón, as well as CI and Brown's vocabulary. Klein, "Klein Technique: Application."

33. Mary Starks Whitehouse, "Physical Movement and Personality: A Talk Given in 1965," *Contact Quarterly* 12, no. 1 (Winter 1987): 16–19.

34. Novack, *Sharing the Dance*, 170.

35. The organization was started in the 1970s by a collective of artists wanting to keep track of a volume of classes happening in the city's privately leased lofts and other independent spaces. Started by Lepkoff, Cynthia Hedstrom, and Mary Overlie, among others, the collective felt that because there was no central organizing body, nothing prevented overlap in the scheduling of classes and workshops. They hoped they could not only remedy that, but also make sure dancers had access to information about what was on offer. Mary Overlie, "(Teacher and Director, Faculty in NYU Experimental Theatre Wing) in Discussion with Author," interview by Doran George, August 6, 2011.

36. Movement Research was initially very similar in nature to *Contact Newsletter*, which is not surprising given the historical proximity of their emergence, and also the involvement of dancers from the same community, such as Lepkoff, who was involved with the start of Movement Research and was a strong proponent of the collective ethics of CI. Ibid.

37. The rapid growth and expansion in Movement Research's New York role exemplifies its professionalism. By 1982, the organization had begun the Studies Project, a series of symposia aimed at raising critical issues; the following year, it began the Open Performance series; and by 1987, Richard Elovich was hired as the first executive director, whose explicit aim was to expand the organization. The operating budget went from $8,811 in 1978 to $160,100 in 1990. "Movement Research Timeline," About Us, Movement Research, last modified 2008–2009, https://s3-us-west-2.amazonaws.com/movementresearch/about/Movement-Research-30th-Anniversary-Timeline-History.pdf.

38. Other 1970s collectives, such as Dance Theatre Workshop (now New York Live Arts or DTW/NYLA) and PS 122, had artistic directors making curatorial choices by the late 1980s. Foster, *Dances That Describe Themselves*, 123. So, to the degree that it validates certain practices, the artistic direction of Movement Research reflects the perspective of a board of artists, much like the content of *CQ* reflects editorial decisions. Furthermore, the publication *Movement Research Performance Journal*, which began in the 1980s, is a mouthpiece through which the more collective nature of Movement Research, compared with DTW/NYLA or PS 122, is represented. The journal has rolling editors addressing various themes that are current for the community and contributors have shared conflicting

opinions even within the same issue, both of which are evidence of the contrast with the single-vision model of an organization with an artistic director.

39. Artists who were teaching Somatics in a way that linked them to the Judson tradition benefited from this cultural capital. Those who got permanent positions include Fulkerson and Cone in the 1970s and Rolland, Kraus, and Karczag in the 1980s. In addition, a large number of artists were employed temporarily throughout the 1970s, 1980s, and 1990s in Europe and Australia.

40. For example, Paxton met Fulkerson while on tour with Cunningham's company at the University of Illinois and subsequently helped her secure her first post at Rochester. His position as an innovator in his own right and member of a revered company were both associated with New York dance and afforded him such influence. It was because of a connection that Fulkerson made with Hassall, at Cunningham's studio, that she eventually became the director of dance at Dartington College in South West England. Fulkerson, "Discussion with the Author."

41. For example, British dancer Mary Prestidge reported in *New Dance Magazine* about an artist in Finland whom she had met in New York. She insisted that reconnection with the artist strengthened each of their artistic resolves to push ahead, despite hostility on home turf. Mary Prestidge, "On the Road," *New Dance Magazine* 16 (Autumn 1980): 12–14.

42. The absence of reference to other contexts as productive of particular ideas in *Movement Research Performance Journal* attests to the fact that the city was not concerned with the discourse of other transnational hubs.

43. Paxton's writing in *Movement Research Performance Journal* emphasizes that artists are benefiting all around the world from the experimentation in New York.

44. The obliviousness of New York to the ideas in other transnational hubs is evident from the way that when Europe achieved significance in the city in the twenty-first century, it was more as a threat to artistic competition in innovation. Once Europe had become a powerful force in the international contemporary dance circuit with the idea of conceptual dance, some of the artists who were associated with the East Village asserted a patriotic insistence that New York had an equal amount of creative innovation. Miguel Gutierrez, for example, ran Young Americans, which was billed as a way to show that "we" can do what the Europeans are doing just as well. And festivals like American Realness showed a consciousness of Europe as a significant artistic force that desires to assert the value in New York's artistic heritage. Gabriela Pawelec, "Tomorrow's Choreographers Danspace Project Brings Together Young Artists in Innovative Dances," *Gay City News*, February 3–9, 2005.

45. The difference between experiments in the early 1960s and the late 1970s is particularly striking in comparing Forti's "Dance Constructions" with Brown's *Glacial Decoy* and Childs's *Dance*, both of which premiered in 1979. I consider these with some depth in chapter 3. For dates of premiers and other details on Lucinda Childs, see "Lucinda Childs Choreography 1963–1989," Choreography, Lucinda Childs Dance, last modified 2019, http://www.lucindachilds.com/choreography-pre90.php#79. For Brown, see "Repertory," Trisha Brown Dance Company, last accessed December 2019, https://trishabrowncompany.org/active-repertory/.

46. Brown cites one 1973 study that found that the back-to-the-landers of the decade were "overwhelmingly white, under thirty, and economically, educationally, and socially privileged families." Dona Brown, *Back to the Land: The Enduring Dream of Self-Sufficiency in Modern America* (Madison: University of Wisconsin Press, 2011), 206.

47. Ibid., 210–11.

48. Guilbaut identifies disagreement within the emerging postwar discourse on liberalism about the role of capitalism. But he points out that, although Schlesinger's *Vital Center* disbanded with the mistrust of large monopolies embodied in F. D. Roosevelt's prewar New Deal, it still paid lip service to Americans' mistrust of unchecked commerce by proposing a mixed economy. Guilbaut, *How New York Stole*, 191.

49. Paxton, Forti, Lepkoff, Deborah Hay, and Lisa Nelson all moved to farms or cabins in rural Vermont and neighboring states, while Bainbridge Cohen relocated to Northampton, Massachusetts, where Stark Smith also ultimately established *CQ*. Goren reports that Forti and Lepkoff retained residencies in New England and New York, which they managed by subletting. They continued to teach and perform in New York along with Paxton, who was a member of the New York dance collective Grand Union. Goren, "Discussion with the Author."

50. Stephanie Skura, who became an important teacher and proponent of Skinner Releasing, associates the nature-based imagery in Skinner's work with the pioneer's location in Seattle, and what is more, Skura herself moved to Seattle to escape the demands of New York life. Skura, "Discussion with the Author."

51. San Francisco's sexualized Somatics body represents a potent contrast to the training approaches that developed almost everywhere else in the network. Artists explored some of the ideas related to the "polyamory" movement and the fetish sex movement in relation to CI and Somatics at 848 Community Space, for example. I have not included it in this study simply because of the lack of resources for the necessary research. However, for more information about this work, *Dance Theatre Journal* has a whole issue devoted to the subject and 848 published a collection of writing called "More Out Than In." Doran George, "Guest Editorial 1: Forget Provocation Let's Have Sex," *Dance Theatre Journal* 25, no. 2 (2013): 1–7; Rachel Kaplan and Keith Hennessy, *More Out Than In: Notes on Sex, Art, and Community* (San Francisco: Abundant Fuck Publications, 1995).

52. Writers such as Linda Tomko and Ann Daly talk about this in their books about the early twentieth century. For example, Isadora Duncan proposed that nature was equivalent to harmony, in contrast with the discord of rapid urbanization that was associated with modernity. Daly, *Done into Dance*, 90–91. Tomko also describes the pernicious effects of urbanization in contrast to rural life. See *Dancing Class*, 1–20. In a related tendency, Jane Desmond points out that in the same era, it was thought that time spent in large, open, green spaces would ameliorate working-class unrest resulting from the newly concentrated labor of industrial life, and that the loss of rural life created nostalgia; for example, animals became part of children's imagery, such as toys, whereas before they had served a function. Jane Desmond, *Staging Tourism: Bodies on Display from Waikiki to Sea World* (Chicago: University of Chicago Press, 1999), 159.

53. Brown, *Back to the Land*, 71.

54. Brown's account of the ideals of back-to-the-landers (Brown, *Back to the Land*, 2011) bears striking similarities with Cynthia Novack's propositions about the values that were important in the CI community. Both communities felt that by opting out, they were staging political activism and engaging in spiritual rejuvenation. Novack, *Sharing the Dance*. Furthermore, Brown argues that the early twentieth-century movement was focused on

the benefits of economic self-sufficiency, and living closer to nature became the emphasis in the 1970s.

55. Brown points to a number of couples who had gone back to the land in previous waves of the movement and published or reissued books in the 1970s, establishing them as icons of the movement. Brown, *Back to the Land*, 205.

56. Paxton, Lepkoff, Forti, Hay, Stark Smith, and Lisa Nelson all continued to perform and teach in New York after basing themselves for some or all of the time in New England. This collection of artists tended to pursue an improvisational rather than set approach to choreography, which emphasized the idea of process and seemed more concerned with the experience of the dancer than set choreography.

57. Paxton developed *Material for the Spine*, which focused on embodying the detail of movement principles often through executing very few kinetic forms, such as his series of rolls. Steve Paxton, *Material for the Spine—Steve Paxton* (Brussels: Contradanse Brussels, 2008), DVD, 4 hours. Forti taught animal movement forms by having students visit the zoo, as she did at the European Dance Development Center, in Arnhem, in the 1990s.

58. Paxton used metaphors from rural activity to explain the way physical principles function in the body. He proposed that students could understand corporeal efficiency by imagining how use of the knowledge of levers and fulcrums could facilitate shoveling earth. I experienced him using these ideas when he was teaching in Arnhem in 1993. The idea that nature is a site at which a basic truth of the body is revealed through animal behavior, weather, and plant growth is a metaphor that was liberally used throughout the late twentieth century. Joan Skinner's lexicon of poetic imagery is another good example. Stephanie Skura, "Releasing Dance: Interview with Joan Skinner," *Contact Quarterly* 15, no. 3 (Fall 1990): 6.

59. Brown cites a 1973 study of back-to-the-landers that dubs them "children of prosperity." Brown, *Back to the Land*, 74.

60. In an email Steve Paxton comments, "12 years of being right under NY's nose and being ignored turned into 45 years of living in a wild splendid place and lots of work, especially in Europe. Go figure." Paxton, Email correspondence. Stephanie Skura, on the other hand, who didn't have the same weight when she left New York, had the opposite experience. Email correspondence, December 3, 2014.

61. Novack argues that *CQ* was a solution at the moment when dancers wanted to protect the integrity of CI by rejecting hierarchical and commercial modes of professionalization that the form had rapidly begun to develop. She argues that dancers' skill set had begun to show marked differences as virtuosity emerged in the form, which seemed to contradict the inclusive ethics of CI. Yet, the first generation wanted to sustain good teaching practice as the community of teachers grew. The use of the journal as a mouthpiece for the pioneers allowed them to exert influence without imposing rules. Novack, *Sharing the Dance*, 82.

62. Ibid.

63. The reach of *CQ* on a national and, to some degree, international level, compared with the local activity to which Movement Research is directed, means that it would have been impossible for the Contact Editions collective to regulate classes and workshops in the same way. Novack also argues that although Contact Editions aimed to avoid the explicit regulation of CI, the pioneers have exerted tacit control, which constitutes a form of regulation. *Sharing the Dance*, 87.

64. Artists associated with the Somatics network beyond New York, like Paxton, Nelson, Forti, Lepkoff, and Stark Smith, all continued to teach and perform through Movement Research.

65. Movement Research also appeared critical of professionalism because when other collective arts spaces established in the 1970s appointed artistic directors, such as PS 122 and DTW, Movement Research remained an artists' collective.

66. Buckwalter, "The Anatomy of Center," 3–8, 37.

67. For example, both Ishmael Houston-Jones and K. J. Holmes, who has had a lifelong career as a CI teacher and performer, attended the workshop, as did Laurie Booth. K. J. Holmes, "(Improviser and Teacher) in Discussion with the Author," interview by Doran George, August 15, 2011.

68. Kraus initially trained in Graham technique before going to Bennington and discovering CI and Ideokinesis. Kraus, "Discussion with the Author." Madden discovered the same techniques as a student at Hampshire College after training in ballet in New York. Madden, "Interview with Artist." With the skills they developed, both dancers joined Brown's company at a time when the choreographer stated she was looking for dancers who could move more naturally. Bales and Nettl-Fiol, *The Body Eclectic*, 160.

69. Madden stayed with Brown's company as a rehearsal director even after she stopped performing the choreography. She became a strong proponent of Klein Technique in her own teaching and also participated in coteaching experiments in the early 1990s between the Klein School and the Trisha Brown Dance Company. Madden, "Interview with Artist." Her choices contrast with Karczag, who worked in educational institutions where she could continue to pursue the ideas in New England Somatics of discovering the potential of many different bodies, particularly those that were untrained. As her student at the European Dance Development Center, between 1992 and 1996, I heard Karczag talk about her interest in dancers working very differently with vocabularies not determined by existing ideas about training and based on their own bodies. Karczag, "Discussion with the Author."

70. Skinner began the exploration that gave rise to Skinner Releasing Technique in her position at Urbana–Champaign, which became a meeting place for Paludan, Fulkerson, Rolland, and Topf. In her position at Rochester College in New England, Fulkerson followed Skinner's example as she developed Anatomical Releasing. Buckwalter, "The Anatomy of Center." Meanwhile, Paxton took up residence as Bennington faculty, in 1970, for the four years that Lisa Kraus was a student there (Kraus, 2011), and Lepkoff began giving Somatics classes at the Five Colleges, including Hampshire and Amherst in the late 1970s (Diane Madden, "(Dancer and Teacher, and Rehearsal Direction with Trisha Brown Dance Company) Interview in Discussion with Artist," Interview by Doran George, May 25, 2012).

71. Alongside the emergence of modern dance, H'Doubler distanced her educational approach from professional performance because she felt that the aims of progressive education embodied distinct ethics. Her focus on exploration as distinct from imitation endured throughout the twentieth century in the rhetoric of university programs that privileged investigation and understanding over success in professional dance. Ross, *Moving Lessons*, 137.

72. Fulkerson subsequently conducted a similar practice at Dartington College in her role as head of the dance program, and the Dutch institutions SNDO, CNDO, and EDDC followed suit to some extent independently and to some extent based on her model.

Fulkerson, "Discussion with the Author." De Groot had already begun to invite visiting teachers to her Amsterdam studio, which was very influential in the development of Somatics in Dutch state conservatory dance education. However, the administrative director of the schools, Hougée, saw the value of bringing practicing artists into the curriculum when he followed De Groot to Dance at Dartington in 1978. De Groot, "Discussion with the Author."

73. Fulkerson recalls that as a graduate at Urbana–Champaign, she choreographed on athletes from her kinesiology class, mixed with dancers from her own department, by using simple movement that she felt was inclusive. At the time, Skinner was still using the images alongside established dance vocabulary, such as pliés, in a similar way to classes being taught in New York through Hawkins and Nikolais's studios. Through her choreographic experiments, Fulkerson separated the image work from conventional dance vocabulary. Fulkerson, "Discussion with the Author."

74. Fulkerson suggests that she was conscious that the training she instituted at Rochester and developed further in the United Kingdom and the Netherlands would not equip students to participate in conventional modern dance companies. Like the ethics that dominated CI in the 1970s, Fulkerson wanted her classes to be open for all abilities of any dancer, rather than based on exclusive training: "We wanted the work to connect with humanity." Fulkerson's methodology shared origins with CI; she discovered the potential of untrained bodies through her cognizance of Judson experiments and, like Forti, had trained with Halprin in the idea that ordinary gestures done with awareness had great aesthetic potential. She consequently related to the New York avant-garde as a center of innovation, yet like CI, her approach was developed at an explicit symbolic distance from professional dance. Ibid.

75. For example, participating in Paxton's twenty-four-hour dance class at Rochester prepared Lepkoff and Woodberry for the rehearsal process that led to the first showing of what became known as CI at the Weber Gallery in New York. Lepkoff, "Discussion with the Author." Also, Kraus, Madden, Petronio, and Warshaw had trained in Ideokinesis and CI in New England colleges before they auditioned for Brown, in whose company they all performed. Kraus, "Discussion with the Author."

76. Madden, "Interview with Artist."

77. Monson recalls feeling a sense of relief at Jacob's Pillow when she was taking CI classes from Warshaw and Madden. Because she was on probation at her dance program due to her weight, and festivals such as Jacob's Pillow gave dancers and teachers the opportunity to explore ideas for their teaching, her experience there showed her that something was possible other than the ideas that dominated her own university dance program. She also recalls taking composition classes with Brown, in which students were instructed to make a dance based on what they had eaten for breakfast or their journey to the class. It was a revelation for Monson that dance could be generated from something other than the codified language of existing vocabulary. Consequently, the festival brought her into contact with a whole new way of thinking about dance in the relative safety of New England but nevertheless connected to the professional dance scene in New York. At Jacob's Pillow, she met Victoria Marks, who was a senior at Sarah Lawrence and suggested to Monson that she go there instead. So, the festivals supported networking that could give students other ways of working through seeking out different approaches. Monson, "Discussion with the Author."

78. Paxton, Forti, Nelson, Lepkoff, and Hay were all teaching in Britain and the Netherlands, in the 1970s and 1980s, when they were living in rural New England. Paxton, in particular, included metaphors from farming life in his teaching. De Wit, "New Dance Development"; Jeroen Fabius, *Talk, 1982–2006: School for New Dance Development Publication: Dancers Talking about Dance, 15 Interviews and Articles from 3 Decades of Dance Research in Amsterdam* (Amsterdam: International Theatre and Film Books, 2009).

79. In the early 1980s, the teachers at the Putney Workshop were joined by British dance improviser Laurie Booth, who had been Fulkerson's student in Devon. Julyen Hamilton and Kirstie Simson also seemed to carry an association of New England because they were focused on improvisation and never performed on the more conventional concert dance circuit but became very well known through the CI circuit.

80. One among many examples of the ways that *CQ* addressed its foreign readership was through reports from the European Contact Improvisation Teachers conference. See, for example, Nancy Stark Smith, "Le European Contact Teachers Conference," *Contact Quarterly* 11, no. 3 (1986): 41–44, and Anon., "Study Lab on CI and Sexuality at the 10th European Contact Teachers conference Amsterdam, 1995," *Contact Quarterly* 21, no. 1 (1996): 63–64. Yet, the only reference I found to Europe in *MRPJ*, during the late twentieth century, was a letter from Steve Paxton urging people to donate to Movement Research because, although a small organization, its importance is demonstrated by the fact that European dancers depend on its creative innovation.

81. Contact Editions published Bainbridge Cohen's book, *Sensing, Feeling, and Action*, based on many articles that appeared in *CQ* and the journal's summer/fall 2002 issue focused on Authentic Movement. An author search for Susan Klein and a title search for Klein in the forty-year history of *CQ* produced not one single article.

82. Within a year, the school established its own company, London Contemporary Dance Theatre, which embodied the official aesthetics and methodology of the institution, which were Graham-based technique and choreography, focused on theme, symbol, and myth. Jordan, *Striding Out*, 1. Strider members included students of Britain's first modern dance training institution, and they were disillusioned when emphasis was directed toward a resident company that was established. Experimentation in the arts, more generally, had drawn interest in the possibilities of dance, and when the contemporary dance school first opened, despite the Graham-based training and compositional approach, students from diverse backgrounds experimented with performance art, sculpture, film, and other media in presentations that flouted the conventions of the concert. See Jordan, *Striding Out*, 13–23, or Judith Mackrell, *Out of Line: The Story of British New Dance* (London: Dance Books, 1992), 18.

83. Richard Alston, who spearheaded Strider, rejected offers to work with London Contemporary Dance Theatre because of their explicit desire to attract ticket-buying, middle-class audiences with dance that was not too shocking. Mackrell, *Out of Line*, 10. Instead, Strider used their publicity to align themselves with a "post-Cunningham generation" of dancemakers. De Wit, "New Dance Development," 142.

84. Through several residencies at Dartington College in 1974, Strider encountered Fulkerson, whose influence on the company is well documented. See, for example, ibid., 94; Jordan, *Striding Out*, 37–38; and Mackrell, *Out of Line*, 20.

85. Fulkerson made a condition of her Dartington appointment that visiting American artists were budgeted for. Choreographers she had brought to Rochester now traveled from their homes in New England and elsewhere to teach at Dartington, along with Fulkerson's artistic colleagues from the University of Illinois, such as Rollands and Nancy Udow. Fulkerson secured support for her to work with Tropical Fruit Dance Company by bringing them to Dartington. Company members included her students from Rochester, such as Lepkoff, Woodberry, and Deborah Chassler. Fulkerson, "Discussion with the Author." Alston recalls the powerful experience of Strider improvising with Tropical Fruit in sessions led by Fulkerson. De Wit, "New Dance Development," 101. Alston became interested in ways of making dances that were not based on the external appearance, while Strider company member Nanette Hassall became interested in the focus on individual development and growth in dance processes. Jordan, *Striding Out*, 38.
86. De Wit, "New Dance Development," 106.
87. Ibid., 123.
88. For example, the term "pedestrian" was omitted, even though it had figured significantly in the initial document. Ibid., 108–34.
89. Ibid.
90. X6 experimentation was ignored or demeaned by the dance press, established dance venues did not program their work, and one of the collective members, who was on the state arts funding subcommittee for dance, reported on hostility toward experimentation. Peter Williams, who was the editor of the powerful publication *Dance and Dancers* and chair of the Arts Council subcommittee on dance, was a vocal opponent of experimentation. Throughout the 1970s, he published articles dismissing the value of artists' investigative initiatives and argued against channeling resources toward those same projects. Ibid., 146.
91. X6 spearheaded "New Dance," which echoed late 1970s British movements toward independence in the other arts driven by innovation in media coupled with an intellectual deconstruction of the history of art forms. Jacky Lansley, "Writing," *New Dance Magazine* 1 (1977): 14. The collective articulated their perspective through classes, workshops, performances, and public discussions hosted at their own studio as well as in the pages of *New Dance Magazine*, which they published for a decade, beginning in 1977. The ideological trajectory and activity of X6 is well documented in Jordan, *Striding Out*; Mackrell, *Out of Line*; and De Wit, "New Dance Development."
92. See, for example, multiple references in *New Dance Magazine* to the idea of working softly with the body, which emerged out of the idea of ease integral to Somatics.
93. Reviews in *New Dance Magazine* of the work of Dartington graduates and listings of their classes and workshops is evidence of the way in which Fulkerson's impact was felt in London, along with the discussion about "release technique" and other Somatics approaches, including CI.
94. Alston spent time studying in New York after Strider disbanded and, on his return, he began choreographing for London Contemporary Dance Theatre and the other major modern dance company, Ballet Rambert, and he also began working with European ballet companies in the early 1980s. Jordan, *Striding Out*, 105–30.

95. The idea that Fulkerson's influence had permeated major dance companies as well as experimental projects was already being put forward in the early 1980s by, for example, Hubbard, who suggested, "through her teaching and performing and those of her students, Fulkerson's gentle aesthetic is quietly permeating mainstream as well as experimental English and European dance." S. Hubbard, "Experimental Dartington Hall Carries on English Tradition," *New Dance Magazine* (1983): 12.

96. Jordan, *Striding Out*, 101.

97. Although Duprès was initially a member of X6, like Butcher, she aligned with what they both called "abstract," rather than political, dance. Duprès distanced herself from X6, eventually leaving the collective to pursue her choreography and perform in work that became understood in Britain as "American Abstraction." Ibid., 80.

98. Ibid., 64.

99. The press often lauded American work presented in Dance Umbrella, while British New Dance was castigated for its poor execution and lack of innovation. Native choreographers working with abstraction were seen by both their colleagues and the dance establishment as emulating American artistic traditions.

100. For example, in the first issue of *New Dance Magazine*, Fergus Early documented where dance funding was being spent, an endeavor he repeated in the publication several times. Fergus Early, "Funding," *New Dance Magazine* 1 (1977): 16–17.

101. Claid argued that innovation had nothing to offer contemporary dance and, instead, emphasized intentional connections with the social, political, and economic conditions of dance making. Innovation signaled abstraction, which Claid argued positioned art as independent from social conditions. Claid initially distanced her improvisatory working process from the physical images in what she called release work. Jordan, *Striding Out*, 68. However, in conversation with me, she admitted that her rhetoric was tied to historical circumstances and that the combination of Somatics and explicit feminist approaches was important in the late 1970s. Emlyn Claid, conversation with the author.

102. Dancers' health and autonomy were directly connected to social circumstances, so although Early and Claid taught ballet, Duprès taught contemporary dance, and Prestidge taught the gymnastics of her movement heritage, they all did so in a way that was influenced by the ideas in Somatics practice. De Wit, "New Dance Development," 147–65.

103. Karczag recalls that she was less interested in X6 precisely because they continued to investigate ballet. On her return to the United Kingdom from the United States, in the late 1970s, Karczag danced with Butcher, who had worked with Summers in New York, in the early 1970s, and introduced formalism and Somatics to the United Kingdom through an independent route from Fulkerson. Butcher's practice predated the New Dance explosion, from which she distanced herself. Along with Butcher, Karczag and other artists who had danced for Butcher, or had an independent interest in Somatics, used the approach in ways that were not dominated by signification. Karczag, "Discussion with the Author."

104. Brown's first appearance on British soil was critiqued as "art in a vacuum" by some *New Dance Magazine* writers, while others used negative criticism in the mainstream press as evidence that the British establishment was out of touch. The contradictory responses reflect the editorial policy of *New Dance Magazine* to entertain diverse perspectives and are symbolic of contradictory opinions within the dance scene about the significance

of Somatics and formalism. David Collins expressed mistrust in the New York abstract dance work, inferring that dance must reveal its social context through explicit political reference. Collins characterized Brown's work as "the 'serious work in a social vacuum' of the New York approach." David Collins, "Review of Dance Umbrella," *New Dance Magazine* 12 (Autumn 1979): 19. Yet, in the same issue, Clare Hayes proposed that people are either in awe of the avant-garde or frustrated with it because the message in the work is not transparent. Her comment reflects the way that artists identified with formalism were interested in the minimalist movement language informed by Somatics, while those who identified with the idea of explicit politics found the work problematic. Hayes also argued that mainstream critics who felt the work was not of the caliber of concert dance did not understand Brown's contemporary practice because they had not followed British New Dance. Clare Hayes, "Review of Glacial Decoy."

105. In the first *New Dance Magazine* editorial, Lansley proposes that a new language is needed to talk about the new dance form, referencing similar strategies in contemporary criticism used in film and theater. Lansley, "Writing and Dance," *New Dance Magazine* 3 (1977): 15.

106. While Lansley insisted a new language of dance must be developed for artists to be able to articulate their projects, Claid critiqued the innovation emphasized in New York Somatics when she insisted there is no new vocabulary and that the only way to move forward artistically is by interrogating the material circumstances within which dance is made and calling to account the political significance of the moving body. Claid's discourse is evident throughout *NDM* in Early's regular updates on the dispersal of public funding for dance. He emphasizes the gross disparity between funding for classical companies and modern dance as well as the channeling of money into large companies rather than independent ventures.

107. Jordan, *Striding Out*, 63.

108. Ibid., 63.

109. Claid notes that in some ways *Dance Theatre Journal*, which first began publishing in 1983, replaced *NDM*, which ceased publishing in 1986. Claid, *Yes? No! Maybe . . .* , 133. The title of the magazine, which was connected to the Laban Center, established a term through which Britain's burgeoning new dance culture could be understood.

110. Ibid., 5.

111. Ibid., 9.

112. This is evident in *Dancing the Black Question*, where Adair talks about community dance. Christy Adair, *Dancing the Black Question: The Phoenix Dance Company Phenomenon* (Alton, Hampshire, UK: Dance Books, 2007).

113. Gill Clarke was a key figure who straddled both sets of ideas and worked in both organizations insisting upon excellence in dance practice while also keenly aware of the problems of the funding and production structures for independent artists.

114. The list of teachers for ID is very long, but some prominent British names include Gill Clarke, who danced for Butcher and Siobhan Davis, as well as Fin Walker, who danced for Butcher and ran her own company. Both women used Alexander and Klein Technique. Meanwhile, Americans included Diane Madden and Susan Klein's teaching partner, Barbara Mahler. "Artists," Independent Dance, last accessed December 2019, http://www.independentdance.co.uk/who/people/teachers/.

115. Rather than training, Chisenhale describes its focus as "artist development, experimentation, research, and the creation of new and exciting dance and movement works." I curated workshops there, in 2001, given by Jennifer Monson and Yvonne Meier. Combining Skinner Releasing with improvisation structures and showings, they were typical of the kind of programming Chisenhale offered. "History," Chisenhale Dance Space, last accessed December 2019, https://www.chisenhaledancespace.co.uk/about/our-history/.

116. In his historical anthology on the school, Jeroen Fabius identifies those that left as "Bianca van Dillen, Krisztina de Châtel, and Yoka van Brummelen . . . the choreographers dominating state subsidized modern dance . . . in the late 1970s and 1980s." He notes that "the school acquired a relatively isolated position," which resulted in it being "a subject of fierce debate in national newspapers." Fabius, *Talk*, 16.

117. For example, Peter Hulton published discussions and interviews that were conducted at the EDDC through the Dartington Theatre papers rubric. Peter Hulton, *Theatre Papers Archive* (Exeter: Arts Archive, 2010).

118. Hawkins encouraged De Groot to interrogate "the nature and mechanics of dance," which she felt contrasted with the focus on fulfillment of form in ballet and Graham technique. Hawkins also exposed De Groot to a broad range of traditions including Bharatanatyam revivalist Tanjore Balasaraswati, Balinese dance, and Flamenco, which she felt opened up greater expressive possibility. Furthermore, while visiting her father in California, De Groot met Halprin through Welland Lathrop, whom she knew from the Limon company. With the exposure to dance ideology influenced by Zen Buddhism, such as improvising on Halprin's outdoor deck in the late 1950s, De Groot felt that there was much greater possibility for creativity than following existing aesthetics. De Groot, "Discussion with the Author."

119. De Groot established her own studio precisely because existing Dutch dance studios wanted her to teach Graham technique, from which De Groot wanted to depart. Ibid.

120. Teachers from within the ballet program wanted to have students do two years of classical training before they trained with De Groot or Stuyf. Ibid.

121. AHK's ballet and modern teachers understood the Somatics approach from Jaqueline Knoops, who was a student of De Groot; De Groot had trained Knoops in pedagogy and asked her to attend the meeting in her stead. Knoops articulated different priorities in De Groot's training of using the pelvis as a center of gravity, moving with ease in and out of the floor, and cultivating awareness of the motion of weight so that the vocabulary of the dance emerged from the directional movement of energy, rather than a predetermined lexicon. She also reported that they worked with percussion rather than a piano during classes to introduce different musical measures including syncopation. Jacqueline Knoops, email correspondence, July 16, 2013.

122. De Groot, "Discussion with the Author."

123. De Groot followed Hawkins's example of embracing broad influences by looking for ideas in experimental theatre, and she also added classes in rhythm and martial arts. She integrated physical, nontextual theater in her studio through the teaching of Jenn Ben-Yakov. De Groot felt that through martial arts students would learn to focus on energy rather than form in their training, which she manifested through the martial arts teaching of Phoa Yan Tiong, later followed by John Yalenizian (Armenia), who taught Tai Chi and

rhythm using an instrument called the "oud" while students would play tin cans or whatever made a noise. Ibid.

124. For a discussion on the history of pillarization and its impact on multiculturalism and Islamophobia, see Marlou Schrover, "Pillarization, Multiculturalism and Cultural Freezing: Dutch Migration History and the Enforcement of Essentialist Ideas [in English]," *BMGN Low Countries Historical Review* 125, nos. 2–3 (2010): 329–54.

125. The breakdown in conversation between Somatics and modern teachers was exacerbated by students' struggle to fulfill both approaches, which was compounded by their experience of the differences between their teachers. Knoops recalls that in meetings to discuss students' progress, conflicting camps emerged, and that while the students expressed the desire for more technique and the modern teachers expressed concern about the lack of physical proficiency, students also flocked to De Groot's classes. Knoops, email correspondence. De Groot, who was still developing her ideas, remembers that she wanted students to have more training than she alone could offer and wanted to be in collaborative dialogue with the Graham and Cunningham teachers. Yet, she also felt that the modern training was counter to her approach. The Graham and Cunningham teachers felt that De Groot's teaching undermined students' physical achievements. De Groot, "Discussion with the Author."

126. Hougée was convinced by Somatics because he felt the Graham teachers were instituting outdated aesthetics in class, like requiring students to shave their armpits and wear no jewelry, and instructing them to smile. The Graham teachers also insisted that dancers must train for years before they could be creative, and choreography was characterized as a predetermined craft along the line of *The Art of Making Dances*, by Doris Humphrey. Hougée felt that Graham pedagogy seemed outdated even for kindergarten. Aat Hougée and Wendell Beavers, "A Search for Words: Providing New Symbols," in *Talk, 1982–2006: School for New Dance Development Publication: Dancers Talking about Dance, 15 Interviews and Articles from 3 Decades of Dance Research in Amsterdam*, ed. Jeroen Fabius (Amsterdam: International Theatre and Film Books, 2009), 50.

127. Teun Voeten, "Dutch Provos," *High Times* 2 (1990): 32–36, 64–66, 73.

128. Aat Hougée, "(Former Director of SNDO and EDDC) Discussion with the Author," interview by Doran George, June 6, 2012.

129. De Groot, "Discussion with the Author."

130. Although Bart Stuyf's work was Graham based, he was not concerned with technique in the way that De Groot or some of the other Graham teachers were, so his position in the leadership did little for the cause of the modern dance teachers. Ibid.

131. It was hoped that Flier, known in the Netherlands as the Dutch Nijinksy, would help resolve the differences after his appointment in 1980. Yet, like Hougée, Flier supported De Groot's approach because he was familiar with developments happening in American modern dance and saw the authoritarian approach to training as outdated. Jaap Flier and Remy Charlip, "Teaching as Learning," in *Talk, 1982–2006: School for New Dance Development Publication: Dancers Talking about Dance, 15 Interviews and Articles from 3 Decades of Dance Research in Amsterdam*, ed. Jeroen Fabius (Amsterdam: International Theatre and Film Books, 2009), 61.

132. Hougée often employed artists who worked on the margins of professional dance by making trips to New York to look at the work being staged in the off-off-Broadway-like

spaces of the East Village. "What I can do through the security of the school . . . is teach artists about their role in society. Telling them 'you are very important,' which does not show through big audiences. You do not have to become popular to be important." Hougée and Beavers, "A Search for Words," 52.

133. Hougée spoke openly about being attracted to the use of theatricality in ways that were aesthetically confrontational. He was attracted to Somatics dancing bodies that seemed to engage in violence and physical risk. Hougée mentioned that he employed the Canadian BMC teacher and dancer Lee Saunders because her publicity material looked wild and confrontational. Other artists he employed, whose work conflicted with 1970s aesthetics associated with Somatics, include Houston-Jones, Meier, Skura, Monson, Jennifer Lacey, Sarah Skaggs, Cathy Weiss, and Jennifer Miller.

134. The publicity for the program stated that students who left the program were expected to work in marginal spaces rather well-funded concert stages.

135. Working at CNDO/EDDC throughout the 1990s and beyond, Karczag's research in her teaching emerged from her experience of dancing Cunningham vocabulary in Strider and performing for Trisha Brown. She felt that even with the innovative vocabulary that Brown achieved with Somatics, the conventional success of the dance company concealed the creative agency of dancers because they appeared as the anonymous tool of the choreographer's vision within large spaces. Karczag, "Discussion with the Author."

136. She saw Paxton perform in the early 1970s at Dartington, of which she recalls, "I had never seen a dancer move in such an ordinary and at the same time extraordinary way. . . . I loved this easy, unmannered way of moving, the intimacy." She regularly talks of "the form of the functioning human body, the elements that fill the form rather than the form itself." Ibid.

137. Thatcher was on the permanent faculty at SNDO as well as CNDO/EDDC. He trained at the Cunningham studio and enjoyed financial support from the Arts Council of England in the late 1970s. Tony Thatcher, "(Choreographer, Teacher, Faculty at Trinity Laban Conservatory, London) in Discussion with the Author," interview by Doran George, September 6, 2012.

138. Thatcher taught students movement in his practice classes, so unlike Karczag, improvisation was not the means by which the body in flux was cultivated. He insisted that set movement could be a vehicle through which dancers could discover the possibilities of their moving selves by letting go of the imperative of success in which the form appeared not to be about the dancers' selves. Ibid.

139. For example, João da Silva, one of the first generation to study at the CNDO, felt under pressure to be less controlled, less formal, and "wilder" in his movement, which he perceived as an imposed artistic agenda in which some faculty wanted something different from what he had to offer. He perceived their desire as a dominant aesthetic that he didn't want to emulate. João da Silva, "(Director of the Artez Academy MFA in Dance) in Discussion with the Author," interview by Doran George, August 26, 2012.

140. Da Silva acknowledges that the aesthetic to which he refers is one that became the dominant expression in the late twentieth century of the Judson lineage, which he came into contact with for the first time at the school. Ibid. The Norwegian CNDO student Sidsel Pape published an article in CQ openly criticizing a dominant school aesthetic.

Sidsel Pape, "Work in Process, Words in Progress: Experimental Dance as Performance," *Contact Quarterly* 19, no. 2 (Summer/Fall 1994): 32–34.

141. For example, 1990s CNDO/EDDC students Tanja Matjas and Rainer Knupp both felt they ought to have access to therapy or counseling. Knupp explained his physical sickness as a result of confusion aroused by the program. Rainer Knupp, "(Feldenkrais Teacher) in Discussion with the Author," interview by Doran George, September 22, 2012. Matjas felt psychotherapy should be integral to a training that was asking students to self-interrogate. (I recall this from being a student alongside Matjas from 1992 to 1996.) The Landelijk Commissie also expressed concern about the intensity of personal experiences that the training aroused for students. Thatcher, "Discussion with the Author."

142. Da Silva insisted that his artistic perspective was valid and used the discourse of experimentation to do so. He critiqued the imposed aesthetic he perceived in the school from the presumption that the aesthetic of the dancing body is something that the student has a role in shaping. Da Silva, "Discussion with the Author."

143. Heggen was a student from 1984 to 1988, under both Rolland and Cone; began teaching freelance at SNDO in 1994; and became full-time faculty in 2008. Gonnie Heggen (former SNDO faculty), email correspondence, June 28, 2013.

144. De Groot, "Discussion with the Author."

145. Trude Cone and Christina Svane, "Back to the Body: Trude Cone Interviewed by Christina Svane," in *Talk, 1982–2006: School for New Dance Development Publication: Dancers Talking about Dance, 15 Interviews and Articles from 3 Decades of Dance Research in Amsterdam*, ed. Jeroen Fabius (Amsterdam: International Theatre and Film Books, 2009), 73.

146. He argued that artists are inflated by professional dance scenes when they provide new languages, but artists are discarded in the period when they are not producing new language, which is untenable. Hougée and Beavers, "A Search for Words," 49.

147. Visiting artists included dancers associated with Dance Exchange in Australia; the X6 collective of British choreographers who investigated the formal potential of Somatics, including Dartington graduates; New York artists from the Judson generation forward, including those who populated the East Village dance and performance art community of the 1980s; practitioners who made their home in New England; Dutch choreographers and teachers, including graduates from the school; and finally artists from other locales across Europe, including performance artists as well as dancers and choreographers. Fabius, *Talk*, 197–99.

148. For example, the Australian theater practitioner Ann Thompson, who was important in the development of Somatics there, first encountered Fulkerson's teaching at the AHK 1980s summer school, which she found out about from *CQ*. Thompson already knew of Fulkerson through Nanette Hassal, with whom she was taking classes in Australia. Ann Thompson, "(Early Teacher of Somatics in Australia) in Discussion with the Author," interview by Doran George, August 20, 2011.

149. It was after he visited the Dartington dance festival that Hougée acquiesced to De Groot's insistence that they should employ artists while they were visiting the Netherlands. Hougée witnessed how the festival functioned as a meeting place for artists in the United Kingdom, other European countries, and the United States and had emphasized New York as the center of innovation. De Groot and Hougée reiterated the model that

Fulkerson had established at Rochester and continued at Dartington. In the 1980s, they began to employ many of the same artists and teachers with whom Fulkerson had cultivated an ongoing relationship through the programs and festivals for which she was responsible. Fahius, *Talk*, 197–99.

150. This was true, for example, for artists associated with Chisenhale Dance Space. It also meant that Fulkerson eventually left the United Kingdom for the Netherlands.

151. Marlou Schrover talks about a "cradle to grave embeddedness" that resulted from pillarization. "Pillarization, Multiculturalism and Cultural Freezing," 332.

152. Hasall and Dumas returned to their native Australia with the explicit intent of disseminating the Somatics ideas and choreographic approaches they had gathered working in the United States and the United Kingdom. Jordan, *Striding Out*, 57. Karczag, who was initially reticent to return full time to Australia, joined them when she was visiting her family and they informed her the company had been state funded. All the dancers had performed in the British company Strider, and when it folded, Karczag went with Alston to New York, while Hasall continued working with Fulkerson for a year at Dartington. Karczag, "Discussion with the Author." Hassall had also previously danced for Cunningham, while Dumas had worked with Trisha Brown, Twyla Tharp, and Sara Rudner, all of whom left a lasting impression on his dancing and his choreography. Ros Warby, "(Choreographer, Dancer, Teacher) in Discussion with the Author," interview by Doran George, January 23, 2013.

153. Hasall was dancing with Merce Cunningham prior to joining Strider, while both Dumas and Karczag had danced with London Festival Ballet, and Dumas went on to perform with Ballet Rambert, Nederlands Dans Theater, and Culberg Ballet as well as Tharp before joining Strider. Karczag, "Discussion with the Author."

154. The company rehearsed, taught classes, and performed in the Sydney Police Boys Club, and also participated in residencies, such as with the Royal Melbourne Institute for Technology, where they lived, performed, and taught. Karczag, "Discussion with the Author."

155. For example, Karczag performed *Soft Verges, Blue,* and *Connecting Passages*, by Alston, and presented collaborative work with the UK dancer and choreographer Miranda Tufnell. Dance Exchange also invited foreign choreographers to present work with them, such as Fulkerson and her husband, Jim Fulkerson, who was a musician and composer that worked for John Cage. Ibid.

156. Hassal and Karczag, in particular, were already committed to Somatics when Dance Exchange first started and had been part of Strider when it lost press and funding support because the company began to use Somatics. Karczag, "Discussion with the Author."

157. Ibid.

158. With a patronizing tone, British writers talked of Strider as a promising project with the potential to mature. Alexander Bland, "Strider Performs," *Observer*, January 20, 1974.

159. They argued that the form may seem remote, but there is something important to be understood.

160. Karczag recalled that Dumas actively worked to engage critics, a venture at which he was very successful. Karczag, "Discussion with the Author."

161. Dumas insisted that Australian modern dance had never flourished because it emulated European achievements to demonstrate its cultural worth. Hassel asserted that while

modern ballet is influenced by modern dance, the exchange does not happen the other way around because modern dance is engaged in risk, whereas ballet perpetuates tradition. Wendy Owen, "Style without Definition," *The Age* (Age Arts), June 18, 1977.

162. See, for example, Mary Emery, "Fair Exchange," *The Australian*, February 21, 1978, and Alan Brissenden, "An Exploration of Body and Space," *The Advertiser*, March 11, 1978.

163. Donne Graves, "The Exchange," *The Catalyst*, May 16, 1977.

164. When Dance Exchange received funding, David Hinkfuss was subsidized to study under Dumas's mentorship, a role that Dumas continued to fulfill by introducing new generations of dancers to practices he had learned from Tharp and Rudner. Dumas continued to use state funding to take dancers to New York, and according to Ros Warby, he became notorious for instilling in dancers that they must go searching. Warby, "Discussion with the Author."

165. Ibid.

166. Only a year after Dance Exchange began, Hassall began teaching at Rusden Teachers College in Sydney, where she implemented Ideokinesis-influenced Anatomical Releasing. Ann Thompson first encountered Somatics through Hassall's student Lyndal Jones, and her recollection of class bears striking similarities to the teaching happening in the United States, the United Kingdom, and the Netherlands associated with Ideokinesis and Anatomical Releasing. She remembers that after working with visual stimuli, such as pictures of the skeleton, and talking about the way in which the structure of the skeleton works and other anatomical information, Thompson and other students would be instructed to lie in constructive rest and work with an image, such as the center line. They would then take the images into movement. Thompson, "Discussion with the Author."

167. Hassall's students, such as Lyndal Jones, began teaching at Melbourne State College (later named Melbourne University College of Education). Jones had recently studied British New Dance in the United Kingdom and began teaching the work she had learned from both Hassall and teachers in the United Kingdom. Elizabeth Dempster also spent time in the United Kingdom after being exposed to Hassall's teaching and went on to teach both with and after Hassall in a program that trained performers at Deakin. A Somatics-focused dance program ran at Victoria University for many years, with teachers such as Elizabeth Dempster. Shona Innes and Eleanor Brickhill were also teachers or students who became dancers. Ibid.

168. A collective of Australian dancers began the journal, in 1986, to address issues that they felt were relevant to their context, which included many of the same issues as the publication's counterparts in London, New York, and New England. For example, in the first issue, Thompson addresses the feminist implications of working with Ideokinesis, which reflects her familiarity with the discourse in *NDM*. Ann Thompson, "A Position at a Point in Time," *Writings on Dance* 1 (1985): 8.

169. Sally Gardner, "Reflections of the State of the Art: A Report on the Small Companies Conference, 1987," *Writings on Dance* 2 (Spring 1987): 12–16.

170. Elizabeth Dempster, email correspondence, February 20, 2014.

171. Unlike the publications in other contexts, *Writings on Dance* was not a register of classes or a forum for diverse community voices heard through letters, reviews, and short opinion

pieces. Rather, it proffered long articles including liberal reference to academic writing from outside of the field as a way to strengthen the credibility of the discourse. Ibid.

172. Thompson, "A Position at a Point in Time," 4–12.

173. *Ways of Seeing* was a British television series that interrogated the meaning in visual culture and was eventually adapted into a book. John Berger, *Ways of Seeing* (London: Penguin, 1972).

174. The artists who developed the fledgling scene in Australia were aware of some of the problems that had been encountered in the United Kingdom, both through direct experience and from reading *NDM*. In addition to the experience of all the Dance Exchange collective members in the United Kingdom, Dempster, who was a key figure in the development of the journal, was also a student of Fulkerson and had danced with Tufnell, Greenwood, and Karczag before returning to Australia. It is notable that throughout the rest of the twentieth century, *Writings on Dance* kept returning to feminism as a framework for thinking about dance. For example, issue three focuses on "Bodies and Power," with the article "Habeus Corpus: Feminism, Discourse and the Body," by Philipa Rothfield, and "Women Writing the Body," by Dempster, while the 1993 issue devoted itself to "Thinking through Feminism," including "Unlimited Partnership: Dance and Feminist Analysis," by Ann Daly; "Revisioning the Body: Feminism, Ideokinesis and the New Dance," by Dempster; "Dancing In and Out of Language: A Feminist Dilemma," by Rachel Fensham; and "Dancing Out the Difference: Cultural Imperialism and Ruth St Denis's 'Radha' of 1906," by Jane Desmond.

175. In 1967, Aboriginal people won full citizenship for the first time in Australian history, and in 1973, legislation was passed that ensured race would be totally disregarded in matters of immigration. The end of the "Whites Only" immigration policy and the introduction of dance funding were both secured by the Gough Whitlam–led government, the first Labor Party to take office in twenty-three years. Joseph Pugliese (Social Justice Scholar, Macquarie University), email correspondence, January 7, 2013.

176. In this sense progressives built upon a history of Australian settlers appropriating native culture to furnish a confident sense of nation. For example, in the 1920s, Margaret Preston shamelessly appropriated Aboriginal design, color, and symbols to produce a primitivist vision of Australian art. Similarly, in dance and music, John Antill's 1930s score and ballet, "Corroboree," represented a romanticized savage-primitive vision of Aboriginal culture with the notion of a unique Australian identity. Massive appropriation of Aboriginal culture with no permission or financial recompense also attended the 1956 Melbourne Olympics and consequent opening up of Australia to international tourism. Meanwhile, Aboriginal people lived under the violence of the Aboriginal Protection Acts, had their children forcibly removed and institutionalized or farmed out as servants or farm laborers, and had no citizenship or civil rights. Furthermore, Aboriginal law, which views the elders as custodians of their symbols, was ignored. Ibid.

177. Aboriginal people reclaimed their expropriated culture through activist politicization of their role in white Australian colonial culture. The early 1970s saw the landmark establishment of the Aboriginal Tent Embassy outside Parliament House in the national capital and the flourishing of Aboriginal political theater, poetry, and other arts as ways of contesting the ongoing colonial regime and its various systems of colonialist representation. Pugliese, email correspondence. In 1972, the Papunya Tula artists group formed and

started transferring Aboriginal sand painting onto canvases and selling them in white galleries. In 1976, Kai Tai Chan formed Sydney's One Extra dance company, which was made up of European, Asian, and Aboriginal Australian dancers. The company explored themes of colonialism with its multiracial cast. Jaqueline Lo, "Dis/Orientations: Asian Australian Theatre," in *Our Australian Theatre in the 1990s: Australian Playwrights*, ed. Veronica Kelly (Amsterdam: Rodopi, 1998), 58.

178. Scott Lauria Morgensen, *Spaces between Us: Queer Settler Colonialism and Indigenous Decolonization*, First Peoples: New Directions in Indigenous Studies (Minneapolis: University of Minnesota Press, 2011), 16.

179. Karczag began performing Brown's choreography in New York in 1979, which was a movement language that seemed to have been born of contemporary innovation. The same can be said for Dumas, who danced for Twyla Tharp and Sarah Rudner while he was in Manhattan.

180. Hassall reports that "[she] had read about the Cunningham Company . . . in one of the American dance magazines. . . . The US was definitely the centre for new dance development. . . . It proved to be a very exciting time to be there." Nanette Hassall, email correspondence, November 22, 2013.

181. Her critique of Klein Technique in *MRPJ* seems like a thinly veiled rejection of its affirmation of professionalism in modern dance and ballet, a set of values that dancers working with Somatics in the 1970s had wanted to disavow.

182. Helen Poynor, working in the United Kingdom, would be a good example of an exception. However, notably, although British dancers know of her Australian roots, this does not figure in her self-description. Helen Poynor, "Helen Poynor," *Walk of Life: Movement Workshops with Helen Poynor*, last accessed December 2019, http://www.walkoflife.co.uk/helen.htm.

Chapter 3

1. Simone Forti, "Young Frog Falls Over," *Movement Research Performance Journal* 18 (Winter/Spring 1999): 14.

2. Meanwhile, contemporaneous work by British artists Miranda Tufnell and Rosemary Butcher reveals that shared ideas flowed between New York and London but were differently framed.

3. The performance was part of a Grand Union organized improvisation festival at a venue on Fourteenth Street in Manhattan. Paxton is unsure of the exact date and location but recalls the performance, which I also heard about from other artists active in New York in the 1970s. Paxton, email correspondence, December 18, 2011.

4. Ibid.

5. During his series of improvised dances, the artist engaged in other forms of preparation including meditating, completing a dancer's barre, and exploring a movement principle. Ibid.

6. Paxton, email correspondence, July 15, 2014.

7. Forti's profound influence on her generation can be inferred from the adoption of her ideas by artists like Paxton and Brown, which is also evidenced in their eventual taking up of the clothes she chose for her dancers. Forti, email correspondence, June 8, 2014.

8. Banes, *Terpsichore in Sneakers*, 28.

9. *Slant Board* was first staged as part of Forti's concert "Dance Constructions" at Yoko Ono's loft in 1961. Virginia B. Spivey, "The Minimal Presence of Simone Forti," *Woman's Art Journal* 30, no. 1 (2009): 13.

10. Made available by the artist. Forti, "Second Interview with Artist."

11. Novack points out that Halprin replaced emulating a choreographer's style with individual movement and argues that Cunningham's dancers were thought not to be working toward a prescribed ideal but training for open-ended possibility. Novack, *Sharing the Dance*, 25–28.

12. Novack conducts a movement analysis of CI articulating twelve styles, many of which share physical aptitudes and communicative intent that highlight the dancer's process similarly to Somatics. For example, "sensing through the skin," "experiencing movement from the inside," "emphasizing weight and flow," and "the dancer is just a person." Novack, *Sharing the Dance*, 115–24.

13. Novack includes photographs captured during CI duets in which the dancer's gaze is invariably lowered, apparently attentive to their own or their partner's physical mass. The images of CI dancers contrast sharply with ones of ballet, modern, tap, and aerobics dancers in Novack's text, which she uses for the purpose of comparison. The dancer's gaze in these other forms is out, toward an imagined or real audience, unabashedly inviting spectatorship. Ibid.

14. Novack herself points to the signifying agency of behavior that appears incidental to the dance when she suggests that dancers "adjust clothing, scratch, laugh, or cough," which, among other things, serves to indicate that they are ordinary people rather than rarified performers. Ibid., 122.

15. Ibid.

16. Novack cites an interview between Paxton and Banes, in which the choreographer defined his project as seeking a way to apply chance procedures to movement generation. Ibid., 54. She further argues that "minimizing control can carry frightening social implications. Disorientation in American social behavior is usually . . . a sign of mental instability, and lack of physical control is generally thought of as a sign of injury, illness, or intoxication." Ibid., 151.

17. Ibid.

18. Morris suggests that in the 1950s universality succeeded against specificity as the appropriate referent for modern dance. Morris demonstrates that in practice, the conceit of universality was in fact the specific, if dominant, white Protestant culture of the United States. Morris, *A Game for Dancers*, 140–43.

19. Novack, *Sharing the Dance*, 68.

20. Ibid., 96.

21. The quote is taken directly from Strider's first application to the Gulbenkian Foundation. Jordan, *Striding Out*, 39.

22. Rachel Fensham recalls that during Strider's residency at the Royal Melbourne Institute of Technology, she participated in long classes that exceeded the conventional idea of training and felt like a participatory performance. Rachel Fensham, "Discussion with the Author," interview by Doran George, November 17, 2014.

23. Jowitt, "Fall, You Will Be Caught."

24. Ibid.

25. Novack, *Sharing the Dance*, 277.

26. Nancy Topf, "Game Structures, a Performance," *Contact Quarterly* 5, nos. 3/4 (1980): 20.

27. Mona Sulzman, "Process as/and Performance," *Contact Quarterly* 4, no. 2 (Winter 1979): 15. Originally printed in *Soho Weekly News* in 1978.

28. Ibid.

29. Topf, "Game Structures, a Performance," 20.

30. Emilyn Claid, *Yes? No! Maybe . . .: Seductive Ambiguity in Dance* (London: Routledge, 2006), 74.

31. Crickmay cites various reviews that focus on bringing the validity of Tufnell and Greenwood's work into question. Chris Crickmay, "The Apparently Invisible Dances of Tufnell and Greenwood (Reprinted from 1983)," *Contact Quarterly* 30, no. 1 (2005): 42.

32. Ibid., 44.

33. Tufnell explains that she "moved more towards the skills developed through release work, Alexander technique, and the T'ai Chi, where the emphasis is on exploring the movement information storied within the body, rather than with more traditional dance skills." Ibid.

34. Ibid., 45.

35. Ibid., 44.

36. Banes, *Greenwich Village 1963*, 205.

37. Ibid.

38. Stephanie Woodard, "Writing Moving," *Contact Quarterly* 2, no. 3 (1977): 16.

39. Banes, *Greenwich Village 1963*, 205.

40. Ibid., 111. Claid, *Yes? No! Maybe . . .*, 100.

41. Gottschild, *Digging the Africanist Presence*, 20.

42. Bill Weber and Davis Weissman, *The Cockettes* (Strand Releasing, 2002), 100 min.

43. Ishmael Houston-Jones learned CI in Philadelphia and became involved in the New York scene in the late 1970s. Houston-Jones, "Discussion with the Author." Meanwhile, Bill T. Jones learned the form from Lois Welk at the State University of New York in Brockport and continued to work with Welk for several years in New England. Novack, *Sharing the Dance*, 75.

44. Houston-Jones recalls that they wrote the list after they had done the dance. Houston-Jones, "Discussion with the Author."

45. "The dancer is just a person" is one of the features of movement style that makes up Novack's analysis of CI. Novack, *Sharing the Dance*, 122. She contextualizes this within the rejection of modernist faith in expressing the human condition on a grand scale. Ibid., 136.

46. The audience laughs when suggestive encounters or missed connections occur as if in acknowledgment that an intimate entanglement between Paxton and Stark Smith does not mean in this dance what it would mean in other circumstances. Pleasure is taken in the embarrassing effort to transform sexual or other significance of the body into one of pure mass and chaste exchange of weight: "We know that when you put your ass in his/her face, it meant nothing like what it would mean outside of this context." Similarly, audience laughter releases tension that is raised by the "missed moments" in the duet. They reassure themselves, each other, and the dancers that failure to achieve what has become the standard technical execution of the form reaffirms unpredictability as an ethical standard of contact improvisation. Jackie Shue, *Contact at 10th and 2nd: Program 2 and 3*

(New York: New York Public Library for the Performing Arts Dance Division, 1983), videocassette, 120 min.

47. Novack points out that dancers generally viewed East Coast CI style as pure compared with the engagement of "theatrical" elements on the West Coast, so when New York artists began working theatrically, it signified a substantial shift. She further points out that the representation of coastal differences did not always reflect dancers' practice. Novack, *Sharing the Dance*, 87.

48. By configuring socially potent behavior as if it were neutral, Channel Z extended a Cunningham-like theory that all movement is dance. For a further discussion of Cunningham's ideas and their relationship to CI, see ibid., 53.

49. Paul Langland, email correspondence, February 19, 2014.

50. The company formed from a group that had been teaching and improvising alongside and with each other in the late 1970s. They wanted to reunite and explore new possibilities. They synthesized vocabularies from the legacy of CI and the influence of Somatics. Ibid.

51. Novack, *Sharing the Dance*, 96.

52. Ibid., 225.

53. For example, Skura recalls that Tim Miller was one of the first people from their milieu to receive press attention and get funding to make work. She remembers that she and Meier and Houston-Jones were shocked that the press represented Miller's work without reference to the whole group because so much of their practice had entailed a collective endeavor and the sharing of ideas. Skura, "Discussion with the Author."

54. Novack, *Sharing the Dance*, 221.

55. Jennifer Monson sensed that having a press pack and engaging in self-promotion were actively frowned upon within her milieu in the 1980s, which included Meier, Skura, and Houston-Jones. Monson, "Discussion with the Author."

56. Neil Greenberg, "(Dancer, Choreographer, Teacher, Faculty at the New School, NY) in Discussion with the Author," interview by Doran George, August 19, 2011.

57. Anna Kisselgoff, "Clash of the Sexes," *New York Times*, December 15, 1988.

58. Ibid.

59. Newson's choreography was supported early on by X6 veteran Emilyn Claid, who commissioned him in 1984 to make work for Extemporary Dance. Claid, *Yes? No! Maybe . . .*, 69. Newson's work extended the imperative of explicit gender critique Claid had worked with in the previous decade, which is clear from the way that Claid writes about Newson's choreography.

60. For a description of the athleticism and use of narrative in *My Sex Our Dance*, see Ramsay Burt, *The Male Dancer: Bodies, Spectacle, Sexualities*, 2nd ed. (New York: Routledge, 2006), 48.

61. *Them* was staged in the East Village space PS 122 that seats between 69 and 128, whereas *My Sex Our Dance* was staged at the Brooklyn Academy of Music that seats between 834 and 3,000.

62. My analysis of the dance is based on observation of DVD provided by Meier.

63. Novack argues that African American social dances that include similar kinds of disorientation influenced the movement culture within which CI emerged, but she does not reference black theater dance forms as contributors. *Sharing the Dance*, 34. See also ibid., 151.

64. Novack specifically cites dance techniques such as "the Lindy," an African American social dance in which women's bodies are regularly inverted, as contributing to the wider movement culture in which CI emerged. Ibid., 34.

65. Dixon Gottschild, *Digging the Africanist Presence*, 4.

66. Ann Cooper Albright insists there was a sea change in CI when dancers moved from pushing for athleticism to engaging different bodies in the mid-1980s, which she attributes to a built-in principle of CI as always looking to open itself to new possibilities. Related moves in early 1990s CI are *Contact Quarterly* focusing on different communities and sexual identity, which actually reflected the broader move within contemporary dance that I refer to in the section on "inventing." Ann Cooper Albright, *Choreographing Difference: The Body and Identity in Contemporary Dance* (Middletown, CT: Wesleyan University Press, 1997), 89.

67. Ibid., 90.

68. Rather than midrange or large concert houses, they performed in art house spaces in large cities with substantial dance communities and artist-run contexts, such as Hothouse, which affirmed the soloists' investigative focus. For example, Eva Karczag performed the dances I focus on later in this section in small, informal, often makeshift spaces in New York, rather than concert houses like the Brooklyn Academy of Music. And similarly in London, she performed in the Place Theatre, attached to the training institution London Contemporary School of Dance, rather than one of the large concert houses.

69. Paxton explains that in 1986 he began working with variations between recordings of the "Goldberg Variations," made by pianist Glenn Gould in 1955 and 1982. He insisted "every time we listen we are different." Steve Paxton and Walter Verdin, *Steve Paxton's Introduction to the Goldberg Variations* (Leuven, Belgium: Walter Verdin, 1992). Burt understands Paxton as working with "the idea of variation and the problematics and paradoxes of live performance that are raised by [Glenn] Gould's recordings." Ramsay Burt, "Steve Paxton's Goldberg Variations and the Angel of History," *TDR: The Drama Review: The Journal of Performance Studies* 46, no. 4 (Winter 2002): 4.

70. Claid, *Yes? No! Maybe . . .*, 74.

71. Jeremy Nelson, who danced for Petronio and has taught internationally, commented that Karczag has the most released body he has ever experienced. He is not alone in his reverence for her physical practice; as someone who was Karczag's student, I have become used to similar reactions whenever I mention her name. Jeremy Nelson, "Discussion with the Author," interview by Doran George, April 1994. In the same year, Australian critic Jill Sykes draws attention to propensities associated with the regimens, such as Karczag's "astonishing lightness and fluency," and suggests "there is no obvious physical effort in her seamless phrasing." Jill Sykes, "Fine Tuned from Head to Toe," *Sydney Morning Herald*, July 26, 1994. Almost a decade earlier, Burt Supree also uses Somatics ideas when he insists it "is intimate wisdom, deep kinesthetic knowledge that Karczag is conveying" in a St. Marks concert about which he remarks "the movement is pure, eloquent." Burt Supree, "Opening the Launch Window: A Juxtaposition of Memory and Sensation," *Village Voice*, October 21, 1986.

72. Speaking about a 1986 improvisation, Burt Supree commented that "the focus of attention is all in the body's relation to itself." Ibid..

73. Agis rethought her use of Somatics due to exhaustion from substantial career success in the 1980s. Agis, "Discussion with the Author."

74. The use of concept by British artists must be understood within a context where Live Art was burgeoning on their own soil and Konzept-Tanz had achieved critical repute in Western Europe. In both cases, discourse revolved around the notion that artistic concept took precedence over the material through which the artists manifested ideas, which in the case of concept dance often meant rejecting recognizable vocabulary, in the work of artists such as Jérôme Bel. I have articulated the ways in which British Live Art and European Koncept Dance intersect elsewhere. Doran George, "Rumpelstiltskin's Contradictory Mandate: The Contemporary Obligation to Weave Cultural Detritus into Avant-Garde Art," in *Inventing Futures: Doing and Thinking Artistic Research with(in) the Master of Choreography Programme of Artez Institute of the Arts, the Netherlands*, ed. João da Silva, Emilie Gallier, and Konstantina Georgelou (Arnhem: ArtEZ Press, 2013), 115–26.

75. Natalie Garrett-Brown, "Shifting Ontology: Somatics and the Dancing Subject, Challenging the Ocular within Conceptions of Western Contemporary Dance (PhD diss., Roehampton University, 2007), 98.

76. Ibid.

77. Meier first staged *The Shining* at PS 122 in 1993 and then again at PS 1 in Queens in 1995. The piece was set in a maze constructed of cardboard boxes, and the dancers led no more than twelve audience members at a time around the space using flashlights. Yvonne Meier, "(Choreographer and Teacher) in Discussion with the Author," interview by Doran George, July 7, 2011.

78. When finally the dancers performed phrases that could be watched, the audience was so close that they were prevented from viewing the spatial design or feats of execution. (My reading of *The Shining* is in part based on my attendance of a reconstruction of the work through Dance Theatre Workshop in 2011 and then again in 2012.)

79. Elsewhere I have argued *The Shining* challenged its audience to participate in the culture cultivated among artists such as Meier, Monson, and Houston-Jones, as well as other East Village artists, such as DD Dorvillier and Jennifer Miller. Many of the dances the performers invited the audience to engage in were based on the artists' own practice. Doran George, "Choreographing New York's Rudeness: Exceptional Behavior in Yvonne Meier's Objectionable Dancing Subjects of the Early 1990s" (Society of Dance History Scholars Thirty-Fifth Annual Conference: Dance and the Social City, University of the Arts, Philadelphia, 2012).

80. Both Valerie Briginshaw and Christy Adair's writing about *Egg Dances* (1988) strongly emphasize the idea that Lee's choreography provides an image of community that has been lost in the modern age of the late 1980s. Christy Adair, "Review of Rosemary Lee's Work at the Place Theatre," *Dice Magazine: The Magazine for Community Dance*, April 1990; Valerie Briginshaw, "'Egg Dances' at the Place Dec. 7th 1988," *Laban News*, Spring 1989. Catherine Hale writes about *Passage* (1990), proposing that the dance represents a forgotten manner of social organization, which it achieves through foregrounding the performer's individual truth. Catherine Hale, "In Rehearsal with Rosemary Lee," *Dance Theatre Journal* 12, no. 2 (2001): 14–17. Even though Lee's work with nondancers was not represented on the stage, the writing about *Egg Dances* (1988/1990) and *Passage* (2001) refers to Lee's community practice.

81. My reading of this piece is based on the documentation provided by *Trisha Brown Early Works 1966–1979, Artpix Notebooks* (Houston, TX: ARTPIX, 2004), 2 videodiscs, ca. 239 min.

82. Sally Banes, "Accumulation Dances," *Chicago Reader*, November 8, 1974, 17.

83. Novack, *Sharing the Dance*, 14.

84. Allen Robertson, "Trisha Brown (Dance)," *Minnesota Daily*, November 15, 1974.

85. Speaking of *Huddle*, which, although first choreographed as part of the 1960 "Dance Constructions," Forti continued to stage throughout the 1970s independently: "She has said that 'it was more placed like sculpture in a gallery space.' She continues to show *Huddle* in situations where 'viewers can be walking around it.'" Carrie Lambert, "More or Less Minimalism: Six Notes on Performance and Visual Art in the 1960s," in *A Minimal Future? Art as Object 1958–1968*, ed. Ann Goldstein (Cambridge, MA: MIT Press, 2004), 105. For further discussion of Butcher's rhetoric, see Chris Crickmay, "Dialogues with Rosemary Butcher—A Decade of Her Work," *New Dance Magazine* 36 (Spring 1986): 11.

86. The works about which I am writing are broadly known as the mathematical pieces. See, for example, Wendy Perron, "Dance Matters: Trisha Brown's Group Forges Ahead without Her," *Dance Magazine*, May 1, 2013, https://www.dancemagazine.com/dance_matters_ trisha_brownaes_group_forges_ahead_without_her-2306908598.html. Brown states her intention was to develop vocabulary within the remit of Rainer's "No Manifesto" and refers to the importance of structured improvisations she participated in with Forti in the documentary about work, *Trisha Brown Early Works 1966–1979*.

87. Banes, *Terpsichore in Sneakers*, 83.

88. Deborah Jowitt, "By Deborah Jowitt," *Village Voice*, April 5, 1973.

89. Banes, *Terpsichore in Sneakers*, 83.

90. Kraus, "Discussion with the Author."

91. Banes, *Terpsichore in Sneakers*, 21.

92. Ibid., 29.

93. Ibid., 31.

94. My analysis of crawling is based on VHS documentation of a 1997 performance in Japan provided by Pooh Kaye. Simone Forti, *Crawling (Tokyo)* (Personal archive of Pooh Kaye, 1976), VHS transferred to DVD. The quotation is from Banes, *Terpsichore in Sneakers*, 31.

95. When she returned to the United States from Rome, where she had begun her animal studies, Forti saw the earliest known fossil remnants of a fish at the New York Natural History Museum in the early 1970s. One of the fins was labeled a "pelvic fin." The idea that an early aquatic animal exhibited nascent human anatomical form convinced Forti that all prior species are integral to human anatomy. She was not aware of Todd's work, despite the obvious connections. Forti, "Second Interview with Artist."

96. Crickmay, "Dialogues with Rosemary Butcher," 10.

97. Ibid.

98. Agis, who danced for Butcher beginning in the late 1970s, recalls "the pedestrian nature was the kind of movement we were all exploring at the time." Agis, email correspondence, February 27, 2014.

99. Ibid.

100. *Glacial Decoy* at New York's Brooklyn Academy of Music. Linda Small, "A Moveable Feast: T.B.D.C. at Brooklyn Academy of Music October 18th," *Other Stages*, November 5, 1981.

101. Ibid

102. Deborah Jowitt, "Postmodern Spectacle," *Village Voice*, November 8, 1983. This is in her 1983 review of *Set and Reset*.

103. Many East Village artists danced in each other's concerts and, much like Crickmay argues about Butcher's practice, sustained a culture in which dancers felt they collaborated on new ideas, in opposition to the model of dancers as interpretive artists executing the choreographer's vision. Like Brown, they built upon 1970s vocabulary even though it moved in a different direction. Monson, "Discussion with the Author."

104. Bedecked in chains, rhinestones, and ostentatious make-up, with lopsided brightly dyed hair, Lauper reconfigured the trappings of conventional femininity toward an image that contested the idea of a compliant woman aiming to attract a man.

105. As chronicled in chapter 1, Kaye, Meier, and some of her other dancers took classes with Ellen Webb, Eva Karczag, and Patty Giavenco, and when Meier began training in Skinner Releasing in the early 1980s, it served her so well in executing the choreography that Kaye asked her to teach some of the company warm-ups. Kaye, "Discussion with the Author."

106. Houston-Jones, "Discussion with the Author."

107. The *No No Scores* described dancing states Monson and Meier found while improvising together, which they used to direct performances into a particular quality while remaining open to impulses by refraining from setting the movement. Meier, "Discussion with the Author."

108. Meier came to New York from her native Switzerland with a government fellowship to study at the Cunningham studio. She felt that despite his rhetoric, Cunningham's company embodied a physical ideal she would never fulfill. Disenchanted by the classes, she discovered CI and Somatics through dancers she met at the Cunningham school. In Webb's classes, CI and Skinner Releasing, she felt there was the potential for much greater artistic freedom and convinced her government that the new approaches in which she trained were more important than Cunningham technique. She had initially been skeptical about improvisation but found she could extend her vocabulary using training in Todd's ideas. Ibid.

109. Colleague Lucy Sexton recalls that the dominant idea on the 1980s left was that lesbian and gay identity should be represented as positive and coherent, preventing more nuanced considerations of queerness. Sexton was part of the East Village duo Dance Noise and worked with Houston-Jones on numerous projects in the 1980s. Lucy Sexton, "(Dance Noise Performer and East Village Cultural Agitator) in Discussion with the Author," interview by Doran George, September 17, 2011.

110. Sandla, "À La Recherche," 22.

111. Ibid.

112. Jennifer Monson, "(Choreographer, Dancer, Teacher) in Second Discussion with the Author," interview by Doran George, April 25, 2014.

113. Jennifer Monson, "(Choreographer, Dancer, Teacher) in Third Discussion with the Author," interview by Doran George, January 13, 2010.

114. Cooper Albright is describing Monson because she is using the work to contrast with the construction in other work of muscular femininity, but her comment applies equally to Jasperse. *Choreographing Difference*, 54.

115. Monson recalls that she was enthralled by televised images of tackling in the 1992 World Cup series. She understood the activity in which players were engaged as movement improvisation. Monson, "Discussion with the Author."

116. The duet was made for the "Sexual ID" series St. Marks Church, and Monson commented that the more explicit themes of identity in the work were Dorvillier's influence, which further attests to the collaborative nature of East Village inventing. Ibid.

117. Houston-Jones also talked about the way the tension he cultivated in *Them* a decade earlier was possible because of sexual dynamics between dancers in the work and those in the East Village community. Houston-Jones, "Discussion with the Author."

118. In a similar way to my argument about how Somatics was used against the patriarchal demands of spectacle, Cooper Albright configures disabled dancers as potentially fracturing the male gaze, both expanding upon and rejuvenating feminism. *Choreographing Difference*, 57.

119. Ibid., 64. In the United Kingdom, New Dance built upon Laban's quiet influence in Britain following World War II. Valerie Preston-Dunlop and Luis España trace the influence in Britain of Rudolf Laban's insistence that dance must be practiced in nonarts contexts. Modern dance was broadly taught as an educational tool in schools in the 1950s, which established its utility as something quite distinct from the art form. Preston-Dunlop and España, *The American Invasion, 1962–1972*.

120. Benjamin formed Candoco with Celeste Dandeker in the late 1980s. Adam Benjamin, *Making an Entrance: Theory and Practice for Disabled and Non-Disabled Dancers* (London: Routledge, 2002).

121. The term "community dance" developed to describe practice in which dancers aimed to create access to the art form for populations who were perceived as being excluded. (See, for example, People Dancing, "About Us," People Dancing: The Foundation for Community Dance, last accessed December 2019, https://www.communitydance.org.uk/about-people-dancing.) Christy Adair chronicles the development of such a perspective in relation to state funding in the late 1970s. Adair, *Dancing the Black Question*, 57.

122. Christy Adair points out that "a focus of the community arts was on developing participation, rather than passive experience of the arts, and this approach matched the [Arts] Council's aim of making education a central focus." Ibid., 87.

123. In site-specific spaces, Lee choreographed numerous works including what she calls "community casts" of 250 people of mixed ages and abilities. Some examples include the ruined Haughmond Abbey, Shrewsbury (*Haughmond Dances*, 1990); Fort Dunlop Tyre Depot (*Ascending Fields*, 1992); the Festival Hall Ballroom (*Stranded*); and the Banqueting Hall at the Royal Naval College, Greenwich (*The Banquet Dances*, 1999). She has continued to make work in the twenty-first century. Rosemary Lee, "(Choreographer, Educator) in Discussion with the Author," interview by Doran George, July 21–29, 2012.

124. Teaching untrained dancers, she found that if she used conventional modern dance techniques, the group quickly became stratified on the basis of different degrees of previous training. She found that students lost what she calls their physicality, which is a kind

of comfort with dancing, if she taught phrases set to music because Lee felt the students got caught up in the cerebral demand of fulfilling the steps. Ibid.

125. Lee has worked with companies of mixed ages ranging from dancers under the age of ten to those over the age of eighty. Ibid.

126. Ibid.

127. Candoco used the Tai Chi exercise push-hands, based on breath, and genteel reciprocity to develop vocabulary between disabled and nondisabled dancers. Benjamin, *Making an Entrance*, 3. The similar use of martial arts by Paxton, Forti, and Karczag is no coincidence because Benjamin sites compositional and training trends beginning in the 1960s as crucial to the integration of disabled dancers into contemporary dance.

128. Benjamin cites CI and Graham technique as underpinning Candoco's work, but he also trained in release technique at Middlesex. Ibid., 14.

129. Cooper Albright, *Choreographing Difference*, 78.

130. Ibid., 77.

131. "Dance boom" is a term that Lee recalls was currency within the New Dance community in the 1980s. Lee, "Discussion with the Author."

132. State-funded dance animateurs in various British regions cultivated local interest in the art form on which Lee depended when she conducted projects based in various British locales. The National Association of Dance and Mime Animateurs (NADMA) was established in 1986, ultimately to become the Community Dance and Mime Foundation (CDMF). NADMA was initially a project funded by the Arts Council of Great Britain, with CDMF becoming a client for annual funding in 1990 (https://www.communitydance.org.uk/).

133. Randy Martin, "Dance as a Social Movement," *Social Text* 12 (Autumn 1985): 16.

134. Skura gave her dancers the prompt "limbs of fury" taken directly from Skinner's lexicon. She also reports that the cue "truncated initiation," which she had worked with for some years before training in Skinner's work, was supported by creative propensities cultivated in Skinner Releasing. She also notes connections with Skinner's work in the cue "always moving on the horizontal plane" because Skinner Releasing entails a lot of "gliding movement." Skura, "Discussion with the Author."

135. Skura's dancer, Brian Moran, wanted to be the dying swan, which she fulfilled by using his dream about her carrying a machine gun while smiling and directing. Ibid.

136. Benoît LaChambre danced in the 1986 version of Houston-Jones's *Them*, and the other dancers had participated in intensive Skinner Releasing classes taught by Skura, as well as trained in CI and Klein Technique. Ibid.

137. She gave directions to individual dancers, based on what she observed of their movement tendencies to generate compelling vocabulary, and followed company members' preferences for trying her prompts as solo, duet, or trio material. The dancers focused on body parts such as arms, legs, or head of fury to see what material it generated, altering the size of the gestures, such as "minimal truncated initiation." Ibid.

138. Jack Anderson, "New York Newsletter," *Dancing Times*, February 1988.

139. Elizabeth Zimmer, "Roll Over Beethoven," *Village Voice*, May 26, 1987.

140. The dancers' divergence from the more receptive use of Somatics is also evident in more contained vocabulary, such as the rapid repetition of arm gestures that opens the first of Beethoven's movements, punching the air manically. The action does not ripple through

the dancers in the way that it does in the other choreographies I have discussed; rather than sensing, Skura's dancers seem to have focused on displaying an outward appearance of shape and form into which they were propelled in the throes of Somatics exploration. Stephanie Skura and Company, *Cranky Destroyers* (Huntington, NY: Inter-Media Art Center Production Co., 1987), videocassette.

141. Zimmer, "Roll Over Beethoven."

142. Skura recalls that the final structure emerged as she pieced the learned movement together with the three movements of Symphony No. 5. Skura, "Discussion with the Author."

143. Cohen-Bull, "Sense Meaning and Perception," 274.

144. Marty Munson, "Roll Over Beethoven: Dance Interprets 5th Symphony," *Cincinnati Enquirer*, October 21, 1990.

145. Zimmer, "Roll Over Beethoven."

146. Jack Anderson, "The Dance: Stephanie Skura," *New York Times*, March 2, 1985.

147. It is pertinent that Jack Anderson insists, "Few ballet or modern dance choreographers would probably ever dream of associating such outlandish movements with Beethoven." Ibid.

148. Jack Anderson, "And the Foot Bones Are Connected to the Funny Bone," *New York Times*, September 4, 1988.

149. See, for example, Unknown, "Stephanie Skura October 22–27," *Cincinnati Footprints* 3, no. 3 (Fall 1990): 23, in which the writer directly references Anderson's *New York Times* reviews.

150. Skura had already received some recognition for humorous multidisciplinary works, which the playful quality of *Crank Destroyers* builds upon. She had a booking agent, Soho Booking, and had received a National Endowment for the Arts grant. But *Cranky Destroyers* is significant because it was the first work in which she used the technique of learning from video. Skura, "Discussion with the Author."

151. Novack, *Sharing the Dance*, 139.

152. Bales and Nettl-Fiol, *The Body Eclectic*, 160.

153. Ibid.

154. By making the link between Brown's staging of femininity, in *Glacial Decoy*, with her staging of a mixed company, I am building upon an argument put forth by Ramsay Burt about the men in *Set and Reset*. I am also arguing that the use of Somatics in displaying is central to the way that Brown achieved her reconstruction of gender. For a detailed discussion of how *Set and Reset* disperses masculinity within its overall composition, see Burt, *The Male Dancer*, 154–58.

155. Ibid., 157.

156. Ibid.

157. Marcia Pally, "To See or Not to See (T.B.D.C. Brooklyn Academy of Music Oct. 20–23)," *New York Native*, November 7–20, 1983.

158. Burt, *The Male Dancer*, 157.

159. Burt explains that Brown wanted to explore beyond undignified and clichéd masculine stereotypes to forge new choreographic possibilities. Ibid., 157.

160. Kisselgoff describes the vocabulary as a synthesis of "Trisha Brown, Merce Cunningham and the mutual support in partnering derived from the technique of contact

improvisation." Anna Kisselgoff, "Hurtling, Hurdling and Whirling near the Edge," *New York Times*, May 18, 1992.

161. Claid observes of Maliphant that "the upward aesthetic of ballet merges with the downward aesthetics of release-based movement" (Claid, *Yes? No! Maybe . . .*, 162), which she calls "feminine qualities on masculine bodies" (160). She goes on to argue that this is one way in which "openly gay/queer self identified performers . . . engage the audience through their play with the conflict between masculine and feminine desire" (169).

162. Burt argues that his approach was influenced by British collaborator and lover Michael Clark, who, unlike Petronio, was classically trained and "deliberately betrayed" the British audiences' commitment to ballet with "symbols of degradation [as] a defiant gesture" toward "a tradition that reinforced a value system which oppressed and abjected gay sexualities." Burt, *The Male Dancer*, 161–64.

163. Ibid., 161.

164. Ibid., 162.

165. Burt argues that modern dance carefully constructed the gender of male dancers as heterosexual because when men's bodies are the subject of display, their claim to male power and heterosexuality is brought into question. Burt, *The Male Dancer*, chapter 1.

166. Foster argues that even while modern dance has historically been one of the most open closets for gay men, the performance of anything but heterosexually constituted masculinity by the male dancer has been difficult if not impossible. Susan Leigh Foster, "Closets Full of Dances."

167. I have previously written about the queer strategies employed by Greenberg, Jasperse, and O'Conner. Doran George, "The Hysterical Spectator: Searching for Critical Identification among Dancing Nellies, Andro-Dykes and Drag Queens," in *Meanings and Makings of Queer Dance*, ed. Clare Croft (Oxford: Oxford University Press, 2017), 83–108.

168. For example, she writes, "up will fly a leg, but at the same time a shoulder will curl in, one part of the rib cage will shake down." Deborah Jowitt, "Conversation Pieces," *Village Voice*, June 2, 1992.

169. Kisselgoff, "Hurtling, Hurdling and Whirling," reviewing the premier of *Full Half Wrong*.

170. Nicole Dekle Collins, "Stephen Petronio," in *Fifty Contemporary Choreographers*, ed. Martha Bremster (London: Routledge, 1999), 189.

171. Cooper Albright, *Choreographing Difference*, 120.

172. *Sololos* and *Locus* were often performed differently in each performance because of instructions given before or during the performance, and it was more efficient to learn the accumulations by following the rules of the work than learning by rote. Yet, the composition of *Glacial Decoy* and *Set and Reset* was set, so the manner in which dancers sustained the principle of performing within a set of conditions was by using Alexander and other techniques in the execution of vocabulary. Shelley Senter affirmed this in an email.

173. After joining the company in 1986, Senter was one of the first to teach the choreography to a repertory company (*Opal Loop* for Ballet Rambert in 1989). She insists that the way in which the movement was conceived shifted from originally focusing on fulfilling tasks to emulating appearance. Senter expanded the use of Alexander Technique in classes using set movement, which she applied to her teaching of the repertory so that rather than aiming to achieve the look of the movement, dancers were asked to question how they

were fulfilling an action. Yet, she recalls that after leaving the company, she was brought back to teach her role in a particular work and later discovered that after she had left, the dancer was asked to look at the video, which is an example of how valuing of the individual embodiment of movement was replaced by the solidification of a particular look that dancers were supposed to fulfill. Shelly Senter, "(Dancer and Teacher) in Discussion with the Author," interview by Doran George, February 15, 2014.

174. Laurel Tentindo, who danced for Brown from 2007 to 2012, confirms Senter's conviction, remarking that she experienced an enormous struggle between what she calls the "authentic physicality" she cultivated with Somatics and the demands of the repertory. Tentindo's experience of such a contradiction is striking in comparison with dancers such as Lisa Kraus and Eva Karczag, who almost thirty years before had experienced Brown's repertory as a container within which to make sense of and develop their work with Somatics. The shift exemplifies how the training went from being a way that dancers achieved creative agency within the choreographic process to a skill set within which they fulfilled existing aesthetics. Laurel Tentindo, "(Dancer/Choreographer/Teacher Formerly with Trisha Brown Dance Company) in Discussion with the Author," interview by Doran George, May 14, 2013. Kraus, "Discussion with the Author."

175. Along with changes in Brown's company and Petronio's integration of ballet, Childs actively pursued classically trained dancers as the century progressed, which is evident in the difference between dancers executing Childs's *Dance 1, 2 and 3* in 1979 and those who reconstructed the work in 2011. The twenty-first-century cast displays the balletic line that comes with the high-effect lifted torso, pointed feet, and full, sustained extension in the arms and neck. Childs transformed her work into a theatrical display of minimalism, whereas in the late 1970s the look of the dancers contributed to her minimalist repudiation of display. I saw the reconstruction on May 7, 2011, at Royce Hall, UCLA.

176. Lionel Popkin, who danced with Brown from 2000 to 2003, recalls that some company dancers were training in ballet, while others, like himself, took a combination of Klein and Alexander Technique. He confirms how Somatics no longer seemed to be integral to the rehearsal process but rather was one training approach that dancers employed to be able to fulfill the demands of the choreography. Popkin, "Discussion with the Author."

177. Senter insists that dancers could move within a set of conditions rather than fulfill a particular image precisely because of the ideas about the body cultivated in Somatics, particularly when they were executing a set form. Senter, "Discussion with the Author."

178. Jennifer Dunning, "Trisha Brown Offers Quiet Contradictions," *New York Times*, March 8, 1991.

179. It is striking that both Kisselgoff and Dunning list the dancers at the end of descriptions of the work, Dunning at the bottom of the page, and Kisselgoff's after the description of each piece, which contrasts with the way that reviewers in the late 1970s and early 1980s drew attention to the dancers' individual embodiment of the material. But both Kisselgoff and Dunning mention Laurie Anderson, who composed the music for *Set and Reset*, and Robert Rauschenberg, who designed the set and costumes for the same work. Ibid.

180. Jeremy Nelson, who danced for Petronio between 1984 and 1992, trained with June Ekman (June Ekman, "(Alexander Teacher to the N.Y. Dance Community) in Discussion with the Author," Interview by Doran George, June 4, 2012). He also pursued the Klein Technique teacher training along with Neil Greenberg. Email correspondence.

181. Stephen Petronio, Facebook message to the author, May 26, 2014.
182. Jeremy Nelson recalls that the choreography "involved a lot of our creative contributions from us the dancers." Although "he didn't really work with open improvisations," the process clearly depended on inventing through, for example, manipulations of [Petronio's] phrase material, or making material around a specific task." Jeremy Nelson, email correspondence, May 26, 2014.
183. Collins, "Stephen Petronio," 189.
184. In Dixon Gottschild's book *The Black Dancing Body*, Doug Varone mistakenly calls Roussève a white choreographer, which he attributes to the movement language. Brenda Dixon Gottschild, *The Black Dancing Body: A Geography from Coon to Cool* (New York: Palgrave Macmillan, 2003), 52. Meanwhile, Roussève recalls colleagues at a festival of African American choreography asking him why he was making white dance. The fact that it was physical aptitudes to which Roussève's critics referred is clear because the dance about which they were talking unmistakably staged black subjects, such as a section in which a black woman in a mammy costume sang "Georgia on My Mind." "David Roussève in Discussion with the Author," interview by Doran George, February 2011.
185. I am referring to Ailey's style, which DeFrantz argues became a signifier of an African American choreography and the staging of black subjectivity on a predominantly white concert stage. Thomas DeFrantz, *Dancing Revelations: Alvin Ailey's Embodiment of African American Culture* (Oxford: Oxford University Press, 2004), 25.
186. "Julie Tolentino in Discussion with the Author," interview by Doran George, April 7, 2014.
187. Christy Adair argues that Phoenix was the first black British contemporary dance company. "Review of Rosemary Lee's Work."
188. Ibid., 175.
189. Roussève, "Discussion with the Author."
190. Jowitt, "By Deborah Jowitt (Eva Karczag)."
191. Yvonne Meier commented that, in the 1980s, "I tried to find a manager without any luck [because] . . . my pieces were mostly on such a big scale that producers shy away . . . [and] my work didn't look very good in video [because it] was built on the output and handling of energy which didn't read on video." Yvonne Meier, email correspondence, July 14, 2014.
192. Ishmael Houston-Jones commented that it was difficult to get a booking agent because, as one of the main agents explained, "Pentacle was better for safe, middle of the road small dance companies than work that was happening downtown." Ishmael Houston-Jones, email correspondence, July 14, 2014.
193. Steve Paxton, email correspondence, July 15, 2014.
194. Karczag, "Discussion with the Author."
195. Perron, "Dance Matters: Trisha Brown's Group."
196. Wendy Perron, "The Body as a Discourse," *Women and Performance: A Journal of Feminist Theory* 6, no. 1 (1993): 43.

Bibliography

Adair, Christy. "Review of Rosemary Lee's Work at the Place Theatre." *Dice Magazine: The Magazine for Community Dance*, April 1990.

———. *Dancing the Black Question: The Phoenix Dance Company Phenomenon*. Alton, Hampshire, UK: Dance Books, 2007.

Adler, Janet. "Body and Soul." In *Authentic Movement: Essays by Mary Starks Whitehouse, Janet Adler and Joan Chodorow*, edited by Patrizia Pallaro, 160–89. London: Jessica Kingsley Publishers, 1999.

———. "Who Is the Witness? A Description of Authentic Movement." In *Authentic Movement: Essays by Mary Starks Whitehouse, Janet Adler and Joan Chodorow*, edited by Patrizia Pallaro, 141–59. London: Jessica Kingsley Publishers, 1999.

Adler, Janet, and Joan Chodorow. "Mary Stark Whitehouse's Papers." In *Authentic Movement: Essays by Mary Starks Whitehouse, Janet Adler and Joan Chodorow*, edited by Patrizia Pallaro, 14–15. London: Jessica Kingsley Publishers, 1999.

Agis, Gaby. "Choreographer, Dancer, Teacher in Discussion with the Author." Interview by Doran George. September 7, 2012.

———. Email correspondence, February 27, 2014.

Alexander, Frederick Matthias. *Man's Supreme Inheritance: Conscious Guidance and Control in Relation to Human Evolution*. New York: E. P. Dutton & Company, 1918.

———. *The Use of the Self: Its Conscious Direction in Relation to Diagnosis, Functioning and the Control of Reaction*. New York: E. P. Dutton & Company, 1932.

Anderson, Jack. "The Dance: Stephanie Skura." *New York Times*, March 2, 1985.

———. *Choreography Observed*. Iowa City: University of Iowa Press, 1987.

———. "New York Newsletter." *Dancing Times*, February 1988.

Anon. "Study Lab on CI and Sexuality at the 10th European Contact Teachers conference Amsterdam, 1995. *Contact Quarterly* 21, no. 1 (1996): 63–64.

Bales, Melanie. "A Dancing Dialectic." In *The Body Eclectic: Evolving Practices in Dance Training*, edited by Melanie Bales and Rebecca Nettl-Fiol, 10–21. Urbana: University of Illinois Press, 2008.

Banes, Sally. "Accumulation Dances." *Chicago Reader*, November 8, 1974, 17.

———. *Terpsichore in Sneakers: Post-Modern Dance*. Boston: Houghton Mifflin, 1980.

———. *Greenwich Village 1963: Avant-Garde Performance and the Effervescent Body*. Durham, NC: Duke University Press, 1993.

Benjamin, Adam. *Making an Entrance: Theory and Practice for Disabled and Non-Disabled Dancers*. London: Routledge, 2002.

Berger, John. *Ways of Seeing*. London: Penguin, 1972.

Bither, Philip. "From Falling and Its Opposite, and All the In-Betweens." *Walker Reader*, March 20, 2013. http://www.walkerart.org/magazine/2013/philip-bither-trisha-brown.

Bland, Alexander. "Strider Performs" *Observer*, January 20, 1974.

Briginshaw, Valerie. "'Egg Dances' at the Place Dec. 7th 1988." *Laban News*, Spring 1989.

Brissenden, Alan. "An Exploration of Body and Space." *The Advertiser*, March 11, 1978.

Brown, Dona. *Back to the Land: The Enduring Dream of Self-Sufficiency in Modern America*. Madison: University of Wisconsin Press, 2011.

Brown, Trisha. *Trisha Brown Early Works 1966–1979, Artpix Notebooks*. Houston: ARTPIX, 2004. 2 videodiscs, ca. 239 min.

Buckwalter, Melinda. "The Anatomy of Center by Nancy Topf." *Contact Quarterly Chapbook 3* 37, no. 2 (Summer/Fall 2012): 5.

Burt, Ramsay. *Alien Bodies: Representations of Modernity, "Race," and Nation in Early Modern Dance*. London: Routledge, 1998.

———. "Steve Paxton's Goldberg Variations and the Angel of History." *TDR: The Drama Review: The Journal of Performance Studies* 46, no. 4 (Winter 2002): 46–64.

———. *The Male Dancer: Bodies, Spectacle, Sexualities*. 2nd ed. New York: Routledge, 2006.

Burt, Warren. "Discussion with the Author." Interview by Doran George. January 25, 2013.

Case, Sue-Ellen. *Performing Science and the Virtual*. New York: Routledge, 2006.

Chatterjea, Ananya. *Butting Out: Reading Resistive Choreographies through Works by Jawole Willa Jo Zollar and Chandralekha*. Middletown, CT: Wesleyan University Press, 2004.

Chisenhale Dance Space. "History." Last accessed December 2019. https://www.chisenhaledancespace.co.uk/about/our-history/.

Chodorow, Joan. "To Move and Be Moved." In *Authentic Movement: Essays by Mary Starks Whitehouse, Janet Adler and Joan Chodorow*, edited by Patrizia Pallaro, 267–78. London: Jessica Kingsley Publishers, 1999.

Claid, Emilyn. *Yes? No! Maybe . . .: Seductive Ambiguity in Dance*. London: Routledge, 2006.

Cohen, Bonnie Bainbridge. *Sensing, Feeling, and Action: The Experiential Anatomy of Body-Mind Centering*. 3rd ed. Northampton, MA: Contact Editions, 2012.

Cohen-Bull, Cynthia Jean. "Sense Meaning and Perception in Three Dance Cultures." In *Meaning in Motion: New Cultural Studies of Dance*, edited by Jane Desmond, 269–85. Durham, NC: Duke University Press, 1997.

Collins, David. "Review of Dance Umbrella." *New Dance Magazine* 12 (Autumn 1979): 19.

Collins, Nicole Dekle. "Stephen Petronio." In *Fifty Contemporary Choreographers*, edited by Martha Bremster, 189–91. London: Routledge, 1999.

Cone, Trude, and Christina Svane. "Back to the Body: Trude Cone Interviewed by Christina Svane." In *Talk, 1982–2006: School for New Dance Development Publication: Dancers Talking about Dance, 15 Interviews and Articles from 3 Decades of Dance Research in Amsterdam*, edited by Jeroen Fabius, 73. Amsterdam: International Theatre and Film Books, 2009.

Cooper Albright, Ann. *Choreographing Difference: The Body and Identity in Contemporary Dance*. Middletown, CT: Wesleyan University Press, 1997.

Corfield, Loraine, Louise Williams, Nancy Topf, André Bernard, and Sally Swift. *The Thinking Body: The Legacy of Mabel Todd*. Piermont, NY: Teachers' Video Workshop, 1999. DVD.

Crickmay, Chris. "Dialogues with Rosemary Butcher—A Decade of Her Work." *New Dance Magazine* 36 (Spring 1986): 10–13.

———. "The Apparently Invisible Dances of Tufnell and Greenwood (Reprinted from 1983)." *Contact Quarterly* 30, no. 1 (2005): 42–45.

Da Silva, João. "(Director of the Artez Academy M.F.A. in Dance) in Discussion with the Author." Interview by Doran George. August 26, 2012.

Daly, Ann. *Done into Dance: Isadora Duncan in America*. Bloomington: Indiana University Press, 1995.

Davis, Bridget Iona. "Releasing into Process: Joan Skinner and the Use of Imagery in Dance." MA thesis, University of Illinois, 1974.

De Groot, Pauline. "(Choreographer and Educator) in Discussion with the Author." Interview by Doran George. September 2, 2012.

De Wit, Mara. "New Dance Development at Dartington College of Arts U.K. 1971–1987." PhD diss., Middlesex University, 2000.

DeFrantz, Thomas. *Dancing Revelations: Alvin Ailey's Embodiment of African American Culture*. Oxford: Oxford University Press, 2004.

Dempster, Elizabeth. Email correspondence, February 20, 2014.

Desmond, Jane. *Staging Tourism: Bodies on Display from Waikiki to Sea World*. Chicago: University of Chicago Press, 1999.

Dowd, Irene. *Taking Root to Fly: Articles on Functional Anatomy*. 3rd rev. ed. New York: I. Dowd, 1995.

Dunning, Jennifer. "Trisha Brown Offers Quiet Contradictions," *New York Times*, March 8, 1991.

Early, Fergus. "Funding," *New Dance Magazine* 1 (New Year 1977): 16–17.

Ekman, June. "(Alexander Teacher to the N.Y. Dance Community) in Discussion with the Author." Interview by Doran George. June 4, 2012.

Emery, Mary. "Fair Exchange," *The Australian*, February 21, 1978.

Fabius, Jeroen, ed. *Talk, 1982–2006: School for New Dance Development Publication: Dancers Talking about Dance, 15 Interviews and Articles from 3 Decades of Dance Research in Amsterdam*. Amsterdam: International Theatre and Film Books, 2009.

Fallace, Thomas D. "Was John Dewey Ethnocentric? Reevaluating the Philosopher's Early Views on Culture and Race." *Educational Researcher* 39, no. 6 (2010): 471–77.

Fensham, Rachel. "Discussion with the Author." Interview by Doran George. November 17, 2014.

Flier, Jaap, and Remy Charlip. "Teaching as Learning." In *Talk, 1982–2006: School for New Dance Development Publication: Dancers Talking about Dance, 15 Interviews and Articles from 3 Decades of Dance Research in Amsterdam*, edited by Jeroen Fabius, 61. Amsterdam: International Theatre and Film Books, 2009.

Forti, Simone. *Crawling (Tokyo)*. Personal archive of Pooh Kaye, 1976. VHS transferred to DVD.

——. "Young Frog Falls Over." *Movement Research Performance Journal* 18 (Winter/Spring 1999): 14.

——. "(Artist, Avant-Garde Luminary, and Teacher) in First Discussion with the Author." Interview by Doran George, May 27, 2012.

——. "(Artist and Teacher) in Second Discussion with the Author." Interview by Doran George. February 18, 2014.

Foster, Susan Leigh. *Dances That Describe Themselves: The Improvised Choreography of Richard Bull*. Middletown, CT: Wesleyan University Press, 2002.

——. "Improvising/History." In *Theorizing Practice: Redefining Theatre History*, edited by William B. Holland and Peter Worthen, 196–213. Basingstoke, Hampshire, UK: Palgrave Macmillan, 2003.

Franko, Mark. *Dancing Modernism/Performing Politics*. Bloomington: Indiana University Press, 1995.

Frieder, Susan. "Reflections on Mary Starks Whitehouse." In *Authentic Movement: Moving the Body, Moving the Self, Being Moved: A Collection of Essays*, vol. 2, edited by Patrizia Pallaro, 35–44. Philadelphia: Jessica Kingsley Publishers, 2007.

Fulkerson, Mary. "(Pioneer of Anatomical Releasing and Key Figure in the Dissemination of Somatics) in Discussion with the Author." Interview by Doran George. May 31, 2012.

Gardner, Sally. "Reflections of the State of the Art: A Report on the Small Companies Conference, 1987." *Writings on Dance* 2 (Spring 1987): 12–16.

Garrett-Brown, Natalie. "Shifting Ontology: Somatics and the Dancing Subject, Challenging the Ocular within Conceptions of Western Contemporary Dance." PhD diss., Roehampton University, 2007.

Gelb, Michael. *Body Learning: An Introduction to the Alexander Technique*. New York: Delilah Books, 1981.

George, Doran. "Choreographing New York's Rudeness: Exceptional Behavior in Yvonne Meier's Objectionable Dancing Subjects of the Early 1990s." Society of Dance History Scholars Thiry-Fifth Annual Conference: Dance and the Social City The University of the Arts, Philadelphia, 2012.

———. "Guest Editorial 1: Forget Provocation Let's Have Sex." *Dance Theatre Journal* 25, no. 2 (2013): 1–7.

———. "Rumpelstiltskin's Contradictory Mandate: The Contemporary Obligation to Weave Cultural Detritus into Avant-Garde Art." In *Inventing Futures: Doing and Thinking Artistic Research with(in) the Master of Choreography Programme of Artez Institute of the Arts, the Netherlands*, edited by João da Silva, Emilie Gallier, and Konstantina Georgelou, 115–26. Arnhem: ArtEZ Press, 2013.

———. "The Hysterical Spectator: Searching for Critical Identification among Dancing Nellies, Andro-Dykes and Drag Queens." In *Meanings and Makings of Queer Dance*, edited by Clare Croft, 83–108. Oxford: Oxford University Press, 2017.

Goren, Beth. "(B.M.C. Teacher) in Discussion with the Author." Interview by Doran George. May 28, 2012.

Gottschild, Brenda. *Digging the Africanist Presence in American Performance: Dance and Other Contexts*. Westport, CT: Greenwood Press, 1996.

———. *The Black Dancing Body: A Geography from Coon to Cool*. New York: Palgrave Macmillan, 2003.

Graves, Donne. "The Exchange." *The Catalyst*, May 16, 1977.

Greenberg, Neil. "(Dancer, Choreographer, Teacher, Faculty at the New School, NY) in Discussion with the Author." Interview by Doran George. August 19, 2011.

———. Email correspondence, September 24, 2013.

Guilbaut, Serge. *How New York Stole the Idea of Modern Art: Abstract Expressionism, Freedom, and the Cold War*. Chicago: University of Chicago Press, 1983.

Hale, Catherine. "In Rehearsal with Rosemary Lee." *Dance Theatre Journal* 12, no. 2 (2001): 14–17.

Harris, Emma. "Black Mountain College: An Introduction." Black Mountain College Museum and Arts Center. Last accessed December 2019. http://www.blackmountaincollege.org/history.

Hasall, Nanette. Email correspondence, November 22, 2013.

Hayes, Clare. "Review of Glacial Decoy." *New Dance Magazine* 12 (1979): 26–28.

Heggen, Gonnie, Email correspondence, June 28, 2013.

Held, David. *Models of Democracy*. 2nd ed. Cambridge: Polity Press, 1998.

Holmes, K. J. "(Improviser and Teacher) in Discussion with the Author." Interview by Doran George. August 15, 2011.

Hougée, Aat. "(Former Director of SNDO and EDDC) in Discussion with the Author." Interview by Doran George. June 6, 2012.

Hougée, Aat, and Wendell Beavers. "A Search for Words: Providing New Symbols." In *Talk, 1982–2006: School for New Dance Development Publication: Dancers Talking about Dance, 15 Interviews and Articles from 3 Decades of Dance Research in Amsterdam*, edited by Jeroen Fabius, 46–56. Amsterdam: International Theatre and Film Books, 2009.

Houston-Jones, Ishmael. "(Choreographer and Artist) in Discussion with the Author." Interview by Doran George. June 6, 2012.

———. Email correspondence, July 14, 2014.

Hulton, Peter. *Theatre Papers Archive*. Exeter: Arts Archive, 2010.

Hurwith, David. "(Dancer) in Discussion with the Author." Interview by Doran George. May 6, 2012.

Huxley, Michael. "F. Matthias Alexander and Mabel Elsworth Todd: Proximities, Practices and the Psycho-Physical." *Journal of Dance and Somatic Practices* 3, nos. 1–2 (2012): 25-42.

Independent Dance. "Artists." Last accessed December 2019. http://www.independentdance. co.uk/who/people/teachers/.

Jordan, Stephanie. *Striding Out: Aspects of Contemporary and New Dance in Britain.* London: Dance Books, 1992.

Jowitt, Deborah. "By Deborah Jowitt." *Village Voice*, April 5, 1973.

———. "Fall, You Will Be Caught." *Contact Quarterly* 3, no. 1 (Fall 1977): 28.

———. "Postmodern Spectacle." *Village Voice*, November 8, 1983.

———. "Conversation Pieces." *Village Voice*, June 2, 1992.

———. "By Deborah Jowitt (Eva Karczag)." *Village Voice*, March 8, 1994.

Kaminoff, Leslie. "Release." *Movement Research Performance Journal* 18 (Winter/Spring 1999): Cover.

Kaplan, Rachel, and Keith Hennessy. *More Out Than In: Notes on Sex, Art, and Community.* San Francisco: Abundant Fuck Publications, 1995.

Karczag, Eva. "(Dancer, Choreographer, Teacher) in Discussion with the Author." Interview by Doran George. August 23–28, 2012.

———. Email correspondence, May 27, 2014.

Kaye, Pooh. "(Choreographer, Dancer, Filmmaker) in Discussion with the Author." Interviewed by Doran George. August 15, 2011.

Kisselgoff, Anna. "Clash of the Sexes." *New York Times*, December 15, 1988.

———. "Hurtling, Hurdling and Whirling near the Edge." *New York Times*, May 18, 1992.

Klein, Susan. "Dancing from the Spirit." *Movement Research Performance Journal* 13 (Fall 1996): 20.

———. "Klein Technique: Application." Klein School. Last modified 2005. http://kleintechnique. com/kt_application.pdf.

———. "Klein Technique: History." Klein School. Last modified 2005. http://kleintechnique. com/kt_history.pdf.

Knoops, Jacqueline. Email correspondence, July 16, 2013.

Knupp, Rainer. "(Feldenkrais Teacher) in Discussion with the Author." Interview by Doran George. September 22, 2012.

Kowal, Rebekah. *How to Do Things with Dance: Performing Change in Postwar America.* Middletown, CT: Wesleyan University Press, 2010.

Kraus, Lisa. "(Dancer, Choreographer, Teacher) in Discussion with the Author." Interview by Doran George. August 1, 2011.

Lambery, Carrie. "More or Less Minimalism: Six Notes on Performance and Visual Art in the 1960s." In *A Minimal Future? Art as Object 1958–1968*, edited by Ann Goldstein, 105. Cambridge, MA: MIT Press, 2004.

Langland, Paul. Email correspondence, February 19, 2014.

Lansley, Jacky. "Writing." *New Dance Magazine* 1 (New Year 1977): 14–17.

Lee, Ilchi. *Meridian Exercise for Self-Healing*, Dahnhak, the Way to Perfect Health Series, 2 vols. Las Vegas: Healing Society, 2003.

Lee, Rosemary. "(Choreographer, Educator) in Discussion with the Author." Interview by Doran George. July 21–29, 2012.

Lepkoff, Daniel. "(Choreographer, Teacher) in Discussion with the Author." Interview by Doran George. August 24, 2011.

Lo, Jaqueline. "Dis/Orientations: Asian Australian Theatre." In *Our Australian Theatre in the 1990s: Australian Playwrights*, edited by Veronica Kelly, 58. Amsterdam: Rodopi, 1998.

Lucinda Childs Dance. "Lucinda Childs Choreography 1963–1989." Choreography. Last modified 2019. http://www.lucindachilds.com/choreography-pre90.php#79.

Mackrell, Judith. *Out of Line: The Story of British New Dance*. London: Dance Books, 1992.

Madden, Diane. "(Dancer and Teacher, and Rehearsal Director with Trisha Brown Dance Company) Interview in Discussion with Artist." Interview by Doran George. May 23, 2012.

Martin, Randy. "Dance as a Social Movement." *Social Text* 12 (Autumn 1985): 16.

Matt, Pamela. "André Bernard." http://www.ideokinesis.com/dancegen/bernard/bernard.htm.

———. *A Kinesthetic Legacy: The Life and Works of Barbara Clark*. Tempe, AZ: CMT Press, 1993.

McCall, Brendan, and Paul Langland. "Body of Work: The Life and Teachings of Allan Wayne." *Contact Quarterly* 23, no. 2 (Summer/Fall 1998): 43–49.

McCauley, Alistair. "Umbrelldom," *Dancing Times*, January 1984.

McKenzie, Jon. *Perform or Else: From Discipline to Performance*. London: Routledge, 2001.

Meier, Yvonne. "(Choreographer and Teacher) in Discussion with the Author." Interview by Doran George. July 7, 2011.

———. Email correspondence, July 14, 2014.

Miller, Jennifer. "(Choreographer, Dancer, Teacher) in Discussion with the Author." Interview by Doran George. July 23–27, 2011.

———. "(Choreographer, Dancer, S.U.N.Y. Purchase Faculty) in Discussion with Artist." Interview by Doran George. August 18, 2011.

———. "(Choreographer, Dancer, Teacher) in Second Discussion with the Author." Interview by Doran George. April 25, 2014.

Monson, Jennifer. "(Choreographer, Dancer, Teacher) in Third Discussion with the Author." Interview by Doran George. January 13, 2010.

Morgensen, Scott Lauria. *Spaces between Us: Queer Settler Colonialism and Indigenous Decolonization*. Minneapolis: University of Minnesota Press, 2011.

Morris, Gay. *A Game for Dancers: Performing Modernism in the Postwar Years, 1945–1960*. Middletown, CT: Wesleyan University Press, 2006.

Movement Research. *Movement Research Performance Journal*. New York: Movement Research, 1990–.

Movement Research. "Movement Research Timeline." About Us. Last modified 2008–2009. https://s3-us-west-2.amazonaws.com/movementresearch/about/Movement-Research-30th-Anniversary-Timeline-History.pdf.

Munson, Marty. "Roll Over Beethoven: Dance Interprets 5th Symphony." *Cincinnati Enquirer*, October 21, 1990.

Murray, Alexander. *John Dewey and F.M. Alexander*. Dayton, OH: AmSAT Books, 1991–92.

Nelson, Jeremy. "Discussion with the Author." Interview by Doran George. April 1994.

———. Email correspondence. February 9, 2014.

———. Email correspondence. May 26, 2014.

Nettl-Fiol, Rebecca, and Luc Vanier. *Dance and the Alexander Technique: Exploring the Missing Link*. Urbana: University of Chicago Press, 2011.

Neuhaus, Bettina. "The Kinaesthetic Imagination: An Interview with Joan Skinner." *Contact Quarterly Unbound*, 2010. https://contactquarterly.com/cq/unbound/view/skinner#$.

Novack, Cynthia Jean. *Sharing the Dance: Contact Improvisation and American Culture*. Madison: University of Wisconsin Press, 1990.

Overlie, Mary. "(Teacher and Director, Faculty in NYU Experimental Theatre Wing) in Discussion with Author." Interview by Doran George. August 6, 2011.

Owen, Wendy. "Style without Definition." *The Age* (Age Arts), June 18, 1977.

Pally, Marcia. "To See or Not to See (T.B.D.C. Brooklyn Academy of Music Oct. 20-23)." *New York Native*, November 7–20, 1983.

Pape, Sidsel. "Work in Process, Words in Progress: Experimental Dance as Performance." *Contact Quarterly* 19, no. 2 (Summer/Fall 1994): 32–34.

Pawelec, Gabriela. "Tomorrow's Choreographers Danspace Project Brings Together Young Artists in Innovative Dances." *Gay City News*, February 3–9, 2005.

Paxton, Steve, and Walter Verdin. *Steve Paxton's Introduction to the Goldberg Variations*. Leuven, Belgium: Walter Verdin, 1992.

———. *Material for the Spine – Steve Paxton*. Brussels: Contradanse Brussels, 2008. DVD, 4 hours.

———. Email correspondence with artist, September 20, 2011.

———. Email correspondence, July 15, 2014.

People Dancing. "About Us." People Dancing: The Foundation for Community Dance. Last accessed December 2019. https://www.communitydance.org.uk/about-people-dancing.

Perron, Wendy. "The Body as a Discourse." *Women and Performance: A Journal of Feminist Theory* 6, no. 1 (1993): 43.

———. "Dance Matters: Trisha Brown's Group Forges Ahead without Her." *Dance Magazine*, May 1, 2013. https://www.dancemagazine.com/dance_matters_trisha_brownaes_group_forges_ahead_without_her-2306908598.html.

Popkin, Lionel. "(Dancer, Choreographer, Faculty in U.C.L.A. Dance Dept.) in Discussion with the Author." Interview by Doran George. February 5, 2014.

Poynor, Helen. "Helen Poynor." Walk of Life: Movement Workshops with Helen Poynor. Last accessed December 2019. http://www.walkoflife.co.uk/helen.htm.

Prestidge, Mary. "On the Road." *New Dance Magazine* 16 (Autumn 1980): 12–14.

Preston-Dunlop, Valerie, and Luis España. *The American Invasion, 1962–1972*. Friends of the Laban Centre, 2005. DVD, 108 min.

Prevots, Naima. *Dance for Export: Cultural Diplomacy and the Cold War*. Middletown, CT: Wesleyan University Press, 1998.

Pugliese, Joseph. Email correspondence, January 7, 2013.

Robertson, Allen. "Trisha Brown (Dance)." *Minnesota Daily*, November 15, 1974.

Rolland, John. *Inside Motion: An Ideokinetic Basis for Movement Education*. Rev. ed. Amsterdam: Rolland String Research Associates, 1987.

Rolland, John, and Jacques Van Eijden. "Alignment and Release: History and Methods." In *Talk, 1982–2006: School for New Dance Development Publication: Dancers Talking about Dance, 15 Interviews and Articles from 3 Decades of Dance Research in Amsterdam*, edited by Jeroen Fabius, 15–34. Amsterdam: International Theatre and Film Books, 2009.

Ross, Janice. *Moving Lessons: Margaret H'Doubler and the Beginning of Dance in American Education*. Madison: University of Wisconsin Press, 2000.

———. *Anna Halprin: Experience as Dance*. Berkeley: University of California Press, 2007.

Roussève, David. "(Choreographer, U.C.L.A. professor) in Discussion with the Author." Interview by Doran George. February 2011.

Said, Edward. *Orientalism*. New York: Pantheon Books, 1978.

Sandla, Robert. "À La Recherche Des Tricks Perdue." *Movement Research Performance Journal* 38 (2011 [1986]): 19–20.

Schrover, Marlou. "Pillarization, Multiculturalism and Cultural Freezing. Dutch Migration History and the Enforcement of Essentialist Ideas [in English]." *BMGN Low Countries Historical Review* 125, nos. 2–3 (2010): 329–54.

Senter, Shelly. "(Dancer and Teacher) in Discussion with the Author." Interview by Doran George. February 15, 2014.

Sexton, Lucy. "(Dance Noise Performer and East Village Cultural Agitator) in Discussion with the Author." Interview by Doran George. September 17, 2011.

Sherman, Frieda. "Conversation with Mary Whitehouse." In *Authentic Movement: Essays by Mary Starks Whitehouse, Janet Adler and Joan Chodorow*, edited by Patrizia Pallaro, 29–32. London: Jessica Kingsley Publishers, 1999.

Shick, Vicky. Email correspondence, February 9, 2014.

Shue, Jackie. *Contact at 10th and 2nd: Program 2 and 3*. New York: New York Public Library for the Performing Arts Dance Division, 1983. Videocassette, 120 min.

Skinner, Joan. *Teacher Training Reader*. Seattle Skinner Releasing Teacher Certification Program, undated.

Skura, Stephanie. "Releasing Dance: Interview with Joan Skinner." *Contact Quarterly* 15, no. 3 (Fall 1990): 6.

———. "(Choreographer and Teacher) in Discussion with the Author." Interview by Doran George. May 13, 2013.

———. Facebook message to the author, November 29, 2013.

———. Email correspondence, December 3, 2014.

Skura, Stephanie, and Company. *Cranky Destroyers*. Huntington, NY: Inter-Media Art Center Production Co., 1987. Videocassette.

Small, Linda. "A Moveable Feast: T.B.D.C. At Brooklyn Academy of Music October 18th." *Other Stages*, November 5, 1981.

Spivey, Virginia B. "The Minimal Presence of Simone Forti." *Woman's Art Journal* 30, no. 1 (2009): 11–18.

Stark Smith, Nancy. "Le European Contact Teachers Conference." *Contact Quarterly* 11, no. 3 (1986): 41–44.

Sullwold, Edith, and Mary Ramsay. "A Dancing Spirit: Remembering Mary Starks Whitehouse." In *Authentic Movement: Moving the Body, Moving the Self, Being Moved: A Collection of Essays*, vol. 2, edited by Patrizia Pallaro, 46. Philadelphia: Jessica Kingsley Publishers, 2007.

Sulzman, Mona. "Process as/and Performance." *Contact Quarterly* 4, no. 2 (Winter 1979): 15.

Summers, Elaine, and Joan Arnold. "Interview with Elaine Summers." New York Public Library for the Performing Arts, 2010. Transcript and Digital Sound Discs.

Supree, Burt. "Opening the Launch Window: A Juxtaposition of Memory and Sensation." *Village Voice*, October 21, 1986.

Sweigard, Lulu. *Human Movement Potential: Its Ideokinetic Facilitation*. Lanham, MD: University Press of America, 1988.

Sykes, Jill. "Fine Tuned from Head to Toe." *Sydney Morning Herald*, July 26, 1994.

Tentindo, Laurel. "(Dancer/Choreographer/Teacher Formerly with Trisha Brown Dance Company) in Discussion with the Author." Interview by Doran George. May 14, 2013.

Thatcher, Tony. "(Choreographer, Teacher, Faculty at Trinity Laban Conservatory, London) in Discussion with the Author." Interview by Doran George. September 6, 2012.

Thompson, Ann. "A Position at a Point in Time." *Writings on Dance* 1 (1985): 8.

———. "(Early Teacher of Somatics in Australia) in Discussion with the Author." Interview by Doran George. August 20, 2011.

Todd, Mabel Elsworth. *The Thinking Body: A Study of the Balancing Forces of Dynamic Man*. New York: P. B. Hoeber, 1937.

Tolentino, Julie. "(Dancer and Artist) in Discussion with the Author." Interview by Doran George. April 7, 2014.

Tomko, Linda J. *Dancing Class: Gender, Ethnicity, and Social Divides in American Dance, 1890–1920*. Bloomington: Indiana University Press, 1999.

Topf, Nancy. "Game Structures, a Performance." *Contact Quarterly* 5, nos. 3/4 (1980): 20.

Trisha Brown Dance Company. "Repertory." Last accessed December 2019. https://trishabrowncompany.org/active-repertory/.

Unknown. "Stephanie Skura October 22–27." *Cincinnati Footprints* 3, no. 3 (Fall 1990): 23.

Voeten, Teun. "Dutch Provos." *High Times* 2 (1990): 32–36, 64–66, 73.

Warby, Ros. "(Choreographer, Dancer, Teacher) in Discussion with the Author." Interview by Doran George. January 23, 2013.

Weber, Bill, and Davis Weissman. *The Cockettes*. Strand Releasing, 2002. DVD, 100 min.

Wheeler, Mark. "Surface to Essence: Appropriation of the Orient by Modern Dance." PhD diss., University of Illinois, 1984.

Whitehouse, Mary Starks "Physical Movement and Personality: A Talk Given in 1965," *Contact Quarterly* 12, no. 1 (Winter 1987), 16–19.

Whitehouse, Mary Starks, Janet Adler, and Joan Chodorow. *Authentic Movement*, edited by Patrizia Pallaro. London: J. Kingsley Publishers, 1999.

———. "C.G. Jung and Dance Therapy: Two Major Principles." In *Authentic Movement: Essays by Mary Starks Whitehouse, Janet Adler and Joan Chodorow*, edited by Patrizia Pallaro, 73–101. London: Jessica Kingsley Publishers, 1999.

———. "Creative Expression in Physical Movement Is Language without Words." In *Authentic Movement: Essays by Mary Starks Whitehouse, Janet Adler and Joan Chodorow*, edited by Patrizia Pallaro, 33–40. London: Jessica Kingsley Publishers, 1999.

———. "Physical Movement and Personality." In *Authentic Movement: Essays by Mary Starks Whitehouse, Janet Adler and Joan Chodorow*, edited by Patrizia Pallaro, 51–57. London: Jessica Kingsley Publishers, 1999.

———. "The Tao of the Body." In *Authentic Movement: Essays by Mary Starks Whitehouse, Janet Adler and Joan Chodorow*, edited by Patrizia Pallaro, 41–50. London: Jessica Kingsley Publishers, 1999.

Woodard, Stephanie. "Writing Moving." *Contact Quarterly* 2, no. 3 (1977): 16.

———. "Experimental Dartington Hall Carries on English Tradition." *New Dance Magazine* 22 (1983): 18–19.

Zimmer, Elizabeth. "Roll Over Beethoven." *Village Voice*, May 26, 1987.

Doran George Biography

Doran George (1969–2017) grew up in the Midlands of England and studied dance at the Hogeschool voor de Kunsten, Arnhem, before focusing in their master's degree on Feminist Performance at the University of Bristol. They became centrally involved in the British live art movement and also worked extensively in movement and dance education for children. After coming to the United States, George continued work as a performance artist, deconstructing sociopolitical categories of identity, building small communities, and cultivating radical practices of intimacy. In tandem with these performances, George edited, with Tessa Wills, a special issue of *Dance Theatre Journal* entitled "Forget Provocation, Let's Have Sex" (2013). Entering the PhD program in Culture and Performance at the Department of World Arts and Cultures/Dance in 2009, they conducted extensive research on Somatics and graduated in 2014, during which time they also published essays in *Meanings and Making in Queer Dance, The Oxford Handbook on Improvisation, The Oxford Handbook on Dance and Wellbeing,* and *Transgender Studies Quarterly.* George then taught courses in LGBT/Gender Studies and in Disability Studies at the University of California, Los Angeles, and in the Department of Dance at the University of California, Riverside. They continued work in live and performance art throughout that time while revising their dissertation for publication.

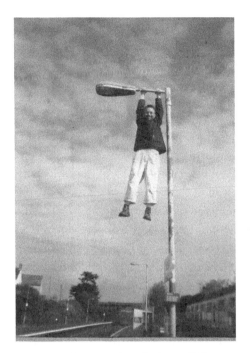

Doran George. Photo by Barry Shils.

Index

Figures are indicated by *f* following the page number

For the benefit of digital users, indexed terms that span two pages (e.g., 52–53) may, on occasion, appear on only one of those pages.

Printed in the USA/Agawam, MA
April 29, 2021

773856.017